Killing Cancer

Julian Lieb, M.D.

ISBN: 1439269076
ISBN-13: 9781439269077
Library of Congress Control Number: 2009913261

DEDICATION

For Lynette and Sarah

I wish to acknowledge the help of Michael Egri and Romain Orlin in the publication of this book.

Contents

INTRODUCTION

The preeminent philosopher of science, Immanuel Kant, pointed out that absolute proof is an illusion. What stands for proof is a hypothesis supported by collateral evidence from various sources. My hypothesis is that antidepressants have anticancer properties, the evidence gleaned from hundreds of sources. Over the past twenty years, I have filed and refiled so many reprints that retrieving and citing them numerically rather than alphabetically would be impossible. However, this is not a textbook or medical journal article, and I ask readers for their forbearance.

To achieve in science, Francis Bacon said, you must practice ethics and charity; and the modern medical establishment answered, "How quaint." Bacon added, "and you must be able to use inductive thinking" and the establishment answered, "No, deductive." Great advances are simple, and emanate from improbable and unexpected sources, said Max Planck, and the establishment answered, "give me one example." Many historians of medicine have noted that while the public believes that advances are made in ivory towers and trickle down to clinicians, the traffic is often in the opposite direction. The establishment replies, "If you spread that around, we'll lose our grants." Loren Eiseley noted that science does not march forward in an undeviatingly line; rather, long periods of stagnation are interrupted by sudden advances. The establishment replies, "We'll have to lay in extra funding for the stagnant years."

On three occasions, I notified the National Cancer Institute of the burgeoning literature on the anticancer properties of antidepressants. Their silence spoke a million words. I notified more than sixty medical schools in the U.S, U.K, Canada, Europe, and South Africa, and they all said, "Get lost." I tried my luck with virtually all the major newspapers in the U.S, Canada, and South Africa, and they gave me the boot. Of numerous literary agents, one proposed that if I changed the book to a diet book, she would find me a publisher. Unqualified gatekeepers for cancer organizations told me that they would read my articles, and decide whether to show them to their medical advisory boards. Of the cancer organizations I approached, only one, a small colon cancer organization, responded affirmatively. While continuing to raise funds, and knowing of the advance, many cancer organizations run modified Ponzi schemes, thus impeding dissemination of the advance. Effectively, safely, and inexpensively preventing or treating cancer is a milestone in the history of man, a great destroyer pacified. Yet in the eight years since I published the first review, thousands of people have suppressed the advance, ethics and altruism cast to the winds.

My sister survived cancer, my mother, seven uncles, and two aunts did not. If I could have them back, most would have survived, and spared the pain, fatigue, and anguish. Antidepressants are not a panacea for cancer, but when effective they switch it off. In "Against Method" Paul Feyerabend noted that suppressing a paradigm in preference for one politically favored could permanently damage society. This is precisely what transpired when venture capitalists and Wall Street launched the genomics bubble, thus rendering prostaglandins orphan molecules. Sages have noted that paradigm shifts do not become medical revolution unless widely disseminated to bypass vested interests. I sincerely hope that many readers of this book will circulate the information to the best of their abilities.

PREFACE

Innovation often has a profound impact on humanity, as the myth of Prometheus illustrates. (Translated by Hugh Rouse):

> "Prometheus was an inventor and filled the earth with animals of his molding, amongst them man. He soon found he could not do much without fire. When Zeus refused to give fire to man, Prometheus tricked him and walked down to earth to give fire. Now he had fire, he began to teach man in earnest. He showed them how to cook, and how to keep themselves warm, how to make bricks, and burn pottery, how to melt metals, and make tools. Men lived no longer in caves and holes in the earth, but made houses to live in. Prometheus taught them how to write, and how to do arithmetic; he taught them about the stars, and gave them medicine to cure their diseases. And they learnt how to tame the horse and the ass and the camel, that these might carry their burdens, and sheep and cows, to give them milk and meat, and to clothe them with skins and fleecy wool. In fact, he taught them the beginnings of all of the arts. When Zeus discovered the deception, he punished Prometheus cruelly; he had him nailed to a rock, while an eagle came and gnawed at his liver; whatever the eagle ate in the day grew again at night. And there Prometheus was left, until long afterwards he was set free."

The gift of foresight may be neutralized by incredulity: The Greek god Apollo vowed to Cassandra, "Yield to me and I will give you the power to predict the future." Cassandra accepted the gift, but reneged when the time came to fulfill her side of the agreement. Apollo allowed her to keep her power, but punished her by decreeing that no one would believe her predictions. Innovators face many problems, as Niccolo Machiavelli noted, "There is nothing more difficult to carry out nor more dangerous to handle, than to initiate a new order of things...partly from the incredulity of mankind, who do not truly believe in anything new until they have had actual experience of it."

Medicine has had its fair share of Cassandra's. The obstetrician Ignace Semmelweiss was ostracized, before his innovation of using antiseptic techniques during childbirth revolutionized obstetrics. Barry Marshall swallowed a brew of bacteria to convince his peers that peptic ulcers are often caused, not by hyperacidity, but by the bacterium, Helicobacter pylori. Earlier, John Lykoudis discovered that the symptoms of peptic ulcer disease and other bowel disorders are often amenable to antibiotics, but no one listened.

In this book, I will provide incontrovertible evidence that antidepressants have remarkable anticancer properties. Once adopted and implemented, the anticancer properties of antidepressants would percolate into every crevice of cancer prevention, treatment, and research. Instead of constantly expanding, the field of cancer would retract; less need for medical, surgical, nursing, and laboratory services; a dramatic reduction in hospital utilization, with a corresponding reduction in energy and water consumption and landfill use.

When a valid treatment model replaces a decrepit one, signs of improvement appear everywhere. Resistance to a new model however, is often so powerful that change can only come about through grassroots activism, widely disseminating the new treatment model, or through political intervention.

Immanuel Kant realized that scientific proof is an illusion. He argued that advances in science consist of inductive hypotheses, strengthened by deductive reasoning. In 1962, Thomas Kuhn described what he called a paradigm, a broad conceptual framework within which many of the detailed answers to particular problems may be found. Paul Feyerabend accepted paradigms as a concept, but argued that they do not traverse the world along rational, scientific lines. Rather, new paradigms invariably become the political victims of an old guard holding onto his power, privilege, and wealth. Feyerabend echoed the insights of Francis Bacon and Claude Bernard. Bacon argued that science is improved by ethics and charity, Bernard that new ideas should be greeted with tolerance. Max Planck noted that advances that are simple, and emanate from improbable and unexpected sources, are those most likely to be resisted. And, in a June 2008 editorial in "Medical Hypotheses" Bruce Charlton exposed "zombie science" as science that died, but keeps returning to life because it serves the needs of wealthy and powerful people and institutions that Charlton refers to as cartels.

One new model meeting stiff resistance is using antidepressants to prevent and treat cancer. The Makerere Medical College in Uganda was the site of pioneering studies on prostaglandins. Prostaglandins are minute, ephemeral, and powerful molecules that self- regulate every cell in the body.[1] At Makerere, Dr. S. M. M. Karim first demonstrated the role of prostaglandins in pregnancy and parturition, while Dr. Williams showed increased prostaglandin levels in the tumors and plasma of patients with medullary cancer of the thyroid. It was at Makerere that David Horrobin and his colleagues began a series of studies on the physiology and pharmacology of prostaglandins. Rashida Karmali, one of Horrobin's graduate students, pursued the role of prostaglandins in cancer while on staff at Newcastle University, the University of East Carolina, and the Sloan-Kettering Institute. She showed that prostaglandin E2 plays a key role in tumor initiation, promotion, and dissemination, with thromboxane B2 involved in invasion, metastases, and the sites of metastases, (thromboxane B2 is a prostaglandin that regulates blood platelets or thrombocytes). Subsequently, Horrobin assembled a team of pharmacologists at the University of Montreal to study prostaglandins. Among their findings was blocking of prostaglandin E2 and thromboxane B2 by tricyclic antidepressants. A paradigm shift was forming, dovetailing with the emerging literature on the antiviral and immunostimulating properties of antidepressants. In 1981, I published the first of nine reviews on the immunopotentiating and antimicrobial properties of lithium and antidepressants. No one has come forward with evidence to repudiate these findings, but thousands of individuals rejected them because they threatened their self-interests.

Cyclooxygenase are enzymes that convert the fatty acid "arachidonic acid" to prostaglandins. Cyclooxygenase -1 (COX-1) is inhibited by indomethacin and ibuprofen. The isolation of cyclooxygenase -2 (COX-2) and the synthesis of selective (COX-2) inhibitors stimulated the pharmaceutical industry's interest in these compounds in preventing and treating cancer, on the grounds that they may have fewer adverse effects than the older, non-selective inhibitors such as ibuprofen and indomethacin. The ability of the latter to prevent or reverse cancer is widely documented, but many are inexpensive. There is no evidence that COX-2 inhibitors are superior to conventional anti-prostaglandin drugs in the prevention and treatment of cancer.

Special interests, many of them corporate rather than medical, largely control the cancer industry. Some exploit such buzzwords as "antioxidants," "diet," "lifestyle" or "vitamins." The observation that Finnish men have a reduced incidence of colon cancer leads to the assumption that their high intake of fiber is responsible. Madison Avenue, and the food and health food industries, duped millions into believing that fiber prevents cancer. The absurd claim that corn flakes "support the immune system" is typical of preying on the helpless.

By the mid-seventies, many studies incriminated prostaglandins in cancer and depression; others showed that lithium and antidepressants inhibit prostaglandins. Were one to spread these articles out on a table, and simply read the titles, the question would arise "Might antidepressants prevent cancer?" Yet to ask that question aloud would raise eyebrows. Relationships that may be obvious to the naïve often elude the sophisticated. A paradigm may fail to emerge not because of successful opposition, but because no one comes forward to champion it, as Thomas Huxley did with natural selection. Philosophers of science have warned that contemporaries seldom promote a rival's success. Researchers may have to do their own marketing, which, according to custom, is not considered civilized. I have waited for almost thirty years for medical schools, hospitals, the pharmaceutical industry, and the medical and lay media to develop and disseminate the antiviral and immunopotentiating properties of lithium and antidepressants. In this book, I will bypass such vested interests in informing readers of the anticancer properties of antidepressants.

A scientific paradox, as defined by Geoffrey W. Hoffman, Julia G. Levy, and Gerald Nepom, exists when there is a conflict between well-supported and widely accepted theoretical dogma or framework and new data, the new data a paradox within the prevailing framework. They argue that many breakthroughs in science were preceded by the emergence of one or more paradoxes; the prelude to what Thomas Kuhn called a paradigm shift. Leonardo da Vinci was fascinated by water, and watched the tiny concentric waves radiate from the spot at which a pebble struck the surface. He assumed, like everyone else did, that he was seeing wavelets. Then it occurred to him that light refraction when the pebble broke the surface tension of the water, created an illusion of wavelets. Albert St. Gyorgy noted, "To see what everyone else has seen, to think what no one else has thought."

According to paleontologist Loren Eiseley, "All of the past generations of men have lived and died in a world of illusions...the simplistic idea that science marches undeviatingly down an ever broadening highway can scarcely be sustained by the historian of ideas. As in other human affairs, there may be prejudice, rigidity, timid evasion, and sometimes inability to reorient oneself rapidly to drastic changes in worldview. The student of scientific history soon learns that a given way of looking at things, a kind of unconscious conformity that exists even in a free society, may prevent a new contribution from being followed up, or its implications from being fully grasped." For more on this, I refer readers to *Stimulating Immune Function to Kill Viruses* (2009, Amazon Books), in particular chapter four, "Depression: The Precursor of Disease" and chapter eight, "Prostaglandins: A Call to Arms."

CANCER

L ife began with the replication of cells; cancer is the accelerated replication of abnormal cells. Thus, the stage was set
for the emergence of both healthy and cancer cells. Cancer cells
grow faster than normal, assume abnormal shapes and sizes, and
lose their ability to function normally. Cancers are usually solid
tumors, but some, like leukemia's, originate in blood forming
organs, and travel through other tissues.

When healthy cells complete their replicative cycle, they
undergo programmed cell death, or apoptosis. Cancer cells are
immortal, and resist apoptosis. A cancer becomes destructive
when its cells enter the blood or lymph streams, and spread to
other parts of the body, (metastasis), where they grow and destroy
normal tissue. Loss of function of essential cells caused by cancer
or its metastases is said to lead to death. I would argue that the
tissues and fluids of patients terminally ill with cancer are as awash
with prostaglandin E2 as to be incompatible with life.

In 1968, Williams and coworkers reported high levels of prostaglandins in medullary cancer of the thyroid. In 1976, Goodwin
and coworkers reported excessive synthesis of prostaglandin E2 in
suppressor T-cells of patients with Hodgkin's disease. Numerous
studies have confirmed elevated levels of prostaglandins in solid
tumors, and in the immune cells and body fluids of cancer patients.
Tens of thousands of studies confirm the role of prostaglandins as
primary factors in causing cancer.

The Causes of Cancer

Many mechanisms are held to cause cancer, some possibly figments of the imagination. They include defective immunity, autoimmunity, viral activation, telomerase activation, apoptosis (programmed cell death), oncogene activation, tumor gene suppression, angiogenesis, and metastasis, accelerated cell replication, signaling disruption, mitochondrial respiration, natural selection, and depression. Excessive synthesis of prostaglandin E2 induces all of them. Should we focus on each mechanism alone, or on the single mechanism responsible for inducing all?

Defective Immunity

Fifty years ago, Sir Macfarlane Burnet suggested that cells of the immune system maintain surveillance for incipient cancer, and if competent destroy it. Factors held to suppress competency include cigarette smoking (lung cancer), chronic esophagitis (cancer of the esophagus), and chronic viral infections (human papilloma virus in anogenital cancers, chronic hepatitis B and C in cancer of the liver, Ebstein-Barr virus in lymphomas). Conventional wisdom holds that chronic inflammatory disorders that predispose to cancer by impairing immune competency include Crohn's disease and ulcerative colitis (colorectal cancer), asbestos exposure (mesothelioma), and excessive sunlight exposure/sunburn (malignant melanoma). Excessive production of prostaglandins predisposes to these disorders, and to cancer, the final common pathway for cancer excessive production of prostaglandins, or deficient production of the enzyme that degrades them.

Autoimmunity

Autoimmunity is the failure of an organism to recognize its own parts as itself, resulting in an immune response against its own cells and tissues. Autoimmune responses are an integral part of immune systems, normally prevented from causing disease by immunological tolerance to the self. In a paradoxical counterpoint to immunosuppression, numerous autoimmune phenomena may occur in patients with cancer. Axiomatically, malignant tumors are diagnosed with increased frequency in patients with such autoimmune disorders as pemphigus, myasthenia gravis, and the Eaton-Lambert syndrome. Prostaglandins have crucial roles in autoimmunity and cancer, but much of the literature on autoimmunity disregards the role of prostaglandins.

Infection

The earliest identification of a virus in human cancer occurred with the association of two cancers with one chronic viral infection. The Ebstein-Barr virus, a member of the herpes family, is linked to Burkitt's lymphoma in eastern Africa, and nasopharyngeal carcinoma in the Orient. Chronic infection with the wart (papilloma) virus is incriminated in anogenital cancer, chronic hepatitis B and C in cancer of the liver. The human T-cell lymphotropic virus type 1 (HTLV-1), is incriminated in adult T-cell leukemia, various cancers are associated with the human immunodeficiency virus (HIV) and members of the herpes virus family are involved in cancer of the uterus and Kaposi's sarcoma.

Viruses have an intimate and complex relationship with prostaglandins. Viruses are harmless unless they replicate, and require sequential fluctuations of prostaglandins to do so. The outcome of contact between a virus, and the prostaglandins that regulate immune function may be death of the virus, its dormancy, or acute or chronic disease and death. The bacterium Helicobacter pylori is incriminated in cancer of the stomach, and the parasites Opisthorcis and Schistosoma haematobium in cancer of the bile ducts and bladder, respectively. Excessive synthesis of prostaglandins depresses immune function, creating vulnerability to these disorders and to cancer, the disorders themselves stimulating prostaglandin production.

Increased telomerase activity

Telomeres are the extremities of a chromosome, their polarity preventing their reunion with any fragment once a chromosome has been broken. Shortening of telomeric DNA is postulated to limit the life span of cells. Activation of telomerase, the enzyme that synthesizes telomeric DNA, is claimed to be an essential step in failed apoptosis and cancer progression. That prostaglandins regulate telomerase is often overlooked.

Failure of apoptosis

Apoptosis, or programmed cell death, meaning, "Falling off of petals from a flower or leaves from a tree" consists of processes leading to the death of a cell. While many anticancer drugs induce apoptosis in cancer cells, they have the same effect on normal cells. Prostaglandins and their regulating enzymes both block and induce apoptosis.

Genes, oncogenes, and tumor suppressor genes

Cancer is often referred to as a "genetic "disease. Cancer cells are said to have such genetic alterations as chromosomal translocations, inversions, deletions, point mutations, amplifications, duplications, or absences of entire chromosomes. Are the fundamental lesions, however, in genes or in the prostaglandins that regulate them?

The oncogene hypothesis suggests that silent or unexpressed "oncogenes" (genes capable of inducing cancer), can, upon proper stimulation, become expressed and thus cause a previously normal cell to become malignant. Silent "oncogenes" are held to be activated by chemicals, radiation, and viruses. Many microbiologists concede that the mechanisms of formation of "oncogenes" and their cancer causing actions are unknown. The literature, however, shows that prostaglandins regulate the synthesis, inhibition and expression of genes, and the growth, differentiation, and replication of cells. Excessive production of prostaglandin E2 causes cancer, genes the variations. Compounds that block the synthesis of prostaglandin E2, such as the non-steroidal anti-inflammatory drugs aspirin, ibuprofen, indomethacin, and antidepressants, arrest cancer, and even reverse it. The clinical effectiveness of non-steroidal anti-inflammatory drugs and antidepressants in numerous malignancies shows that cancer is not a hundred diseases, but one disease with a hundred variations.

Angiogenesis and Metastasis

Tumor angiogenesis is held to be the proliferation of a network of blood vessels that penetrates into cancerous growths, supplying nutrients and oxygen and removing waste products. Tumor angiogenesis is said to start with cancer cells releasing molecules that send signals to surrounding normal tissue, thus activating genes that make proteins grow new blood vessels. Vascularization is said to enhance the aggression of a tumor, by transporting an increased supply of nutrients to it, and favoring progressively more malignant cells.

In 1983, Rashida Karmali showed that prostaglandins and thromboxanes induce cancer initiation, promotion, and metastasis.

She found that the concentrations of thromboxanes in human breast cancer specimens are associated with three clinical variables—tumor size, axillary lymph node metastases, and distant metastases. She suggested that the mechanisms in which prostaglandins and thromboxanes induce metastasis include induction of protein-destroying enzyme production, neovascularization, and subversion of immune function. Metastasis involves the adherence of circulating tumor cells to endothelial cells or to basement membranes, with local tissue concentrations of thromboxanes determining the sites of metastasis. Is there a difference between Karmali's neovascularization and the vascularization central to the angiogenesis theory?

Signaling

Signal transduction involves the conversion by a cell of one kind of signal to another. Most processes of signal transduction involve sequences of reactions carried out by enzymes and activated by second messengers. These processes are often rapid, but may take days to complete. A small stimulus resulting in a large reaction is referred to as amplification of the signal.

Prostaglandins perform a multitude of signaling functions. That they are soluble in fat, and can cross biological membranes, are prerequisites for such actions. Numerous signaling defects in activating and inactivating genes, proteins, and enzymes are involved in cancer, the involvement of prostaglandins often ignored.

Accelerated Cell Replication

In 1981, Armato and Andreis showed that arachidonic acid stimulates the DNA-synthesizing and cell division activities of liver cells. In 1983, they reported that prostaglandins intensely stimulate these activities. In 1990, Goodlad reported that the increase in gastric mucosal mass induced by a synthetic prostaglandin analog, in the stomach of dogs is due to increased cell production. The increase was the result of a dramatic increase in the surface mucous cells.

Mitochondrial Dysfunction

Mitochondria are organelles that take in nutrients, break them down, and create energy, a process known as cellular respiration. Some cells have one mitochondrion, others thousands.

Over seventy years ago, Otto Warburg theorized that a key event in cancer involved injury to the respiratory machinery, resulting in compensatory increases in the utilization of glucose rather than oxygen for energy. Warburg speculated that differences in energy metabolism between normal and cancer cells might offer an opportunity to kill cancer while sparing healthy ones. The mitochondrial alterations that underlie the increased dependence of cancer cells on the aerobic utilization of glucose for energy are held to be a mystery by those unaware of the regulation of mitochondria by prostaglandins. Compounds identified as activating mitochondria (mitocans) include antidepressants, and target the mitochondria of cancer cells, while sparing those of healthy ones.

Excessive Production of Prostaglandins

Prostaglandins were first incriminated in cancer in 1986, subsequently supported by tens of thousands of studies. In the 1970s, antidepressants were shown to oppose prostaglandins. Tragically, the relationship of these bodies of knowledge to each other was not recognized.

Such prostaglandin-synthesis inhibitors as indomethacin and ibuprofen can induce regression of colon polyps. Chronic use of such prostaglandin synthesis inhibitors, like aspirin and ibuprofen, has reduced the risk of colon cancer by as much as fifty per cent. Chronic use of aspirin significantly improves survival in patients with non-metastatic colorectal cancer. Prostaglandin synthesis inhibitors have regressed the skin cancer known as xeroderma pigmentosa, and the lung metastases of uterine cancer.

The isolation of cyclooxygenase-2 (COX-2) and the synthesis of selective COX-2 inhibitors such as Vioxx and Celebrex stimulated research into this enzyme in cancer, and its role in apoptosis. COX-2 over expression inhibits apoptosis. COX-2 is up regulated in such cancers as those of the head and neck, breast, lung, pancreas, bladder, cervix, prostate and mesothelium.

Were it not for their low cost, aspirin, ibuprofen, and indomethacin would have achieved a larger role in preventing and treating cancer than they have.

Natural Selection

Charles Darwin referred to a force in nature favoring reproduction over fertility, and survival over extinction, as natural selection, the primary factor in evolution. In their landmark study on infertility published in 1930, Rafael Kurzrok and Charles Lieb identified factors in semen and uteri that differentiate between fertility and infertility. These factors were later extracted from the semen of boars and labeled prostaglandins, because small quantities of them were found in the prostate. When every cell in the body was found to produce these molecules, it was too late. The name was irreversibly entrenched in the biomedical literature.

Prostaglandins determine whether we are healthy or develop depression, cancer, heart disease, infectious disorders, osteoporosis, neurovegetative disorders, diabetes, obesity, and many other conditions favoring death and extinction. Every cell that differentiates between fertility and infertility, and between survival and extinction, contributes to natural selection, and prostaglandins regulate all of these cells. What Darwin referred to as natural selection, and prostaglandins, are one and the same.

Depression: A Precursor of Cancer

In the Ward Jones lecture given at Manchester University in 1957, Sir Heneage Ogilvie commented, "I have slowly come to frame in my mind an aphorism that can never be stated as such, because no statistics can be advanced to support it: 'The happy man never gets cancer'.... The instances where the first recognizable onset of cancer has followed almost immediately on some disaster, bereavement, the breakup of a relationship, a financial crisis, or an accident are so numerous that they suggest that some controlling force that has hitherto kept the outbreak...in check has been removed."

In 1998, B. W. J. H Penninx and her coworkers at the National Institute of Aging provided compelling evidence for Ogilvie's hypothesis: Chronically depressed people over the age of seventy are eighty-eight per cent more likely to develop cancer, and twice as likely to die of it as their cheerful peers.

The Environment

Cancer may be induced by an identifiable environmental factor such as ionizing radiation, tobacco smoke, or such viruses as hepatitis B and C. All induce prostaglandin E2. Conversely, internal factors, such as defective immunity or aging, may be the culprit. Prostaglandin E2 steadily increases with age, and may be the cause of aging. This would explain why many disorders caused by prostaglandin E2 increase with aging. Whenever the synthesis of prostaglandins is up regulated or their degradation down-regulated, the metabolic environment for cancer comes into play.

References

Abdulla Y. H., Hamadah K. Effect of ADP on prostaglandin E1 formation in blood platelets from patients with depression, mania and schizophrenia. Br. J. Psychiatry 1975; 127: 591-95.

Achiwa H., Yatabe Y., Hida T. et al. Prognostic significance of elevated cyclooxygenase-2 expression in primary, resected lung adenocarcinomas. Clin. Cancer Res. 1999; 5(5): 1001-5.

Ali B. H., Bartlet A. L. Inhibition of monoamine oxidase in chickens and ducklings by a microbial metabolite of furazolidone. Q. J. Exp. Physiol. 1982; 67:69-79.

Al-Saleem T. Skin cancers in xeroderma pigmentosum: Response to indomethacin and steroids. Lancet 1980; 264-66.

Amlot P. L., Chivers A., Heizelmann D., Youlten L. J. F. Increased prostaglandin synthesis in Hodgkin's disease: A lymphocyte-monocyte interaction. Adv. Prost. Thromb. Res. 1980; 6:529-32.

Amsterdam J. D., Maislin G., Rybakowski J. A possible antiviral action of lithium carbonate in herpes simplex virus infections. Biol. Psychiatry 1990; 27:447-53.

Ansell D., Belch J. J., Forbes C. D. Depression and prostacyclin infusion. Lancet 1986; 2:1203-05.

Armato U., Andreis P. G. Prostaglandins of the F series are extremely powerful growth factors for primary neonatal rat hepatocytes. Life Sci. 1983; 33:1745-55.

Balch C. M., Dougherty P. A., Tilden, A. B. Excessive prostaglandin E2 production by suppressor monocytes in head and neck cancer patients. Ann. Surg. 1982 Dec; 645-50.

Baliff B. A., Mincek N. V., Barratt J. T., et al. Interaction of cyclooxygenases with an apoptosis- and autoimmunity-associated protein. Proc. Natl. Acad. Sci. USA 1996; 93: 5544-49.

Bennett A., Carter R. L., Stamford I. F., Tanner, N. S. B. Prostaglandin-like material extracted from squamous carcinomas of the head and neck. Br. J. Cancer 1980; 41:204-9.

Bennett A., Houghton J., Leaper D. J., Stamford I. F. Cancer growth, response to treatment and survival time in mice: Beneficial effect of the prostaglandin synthesis inhibitor flurbiprofen. Prostaglandins Feb 1979; 17(2):179-91.

Bennett A., Berstock D. A., Harris M., Raja B., Rowe D. J. F. Prostaglandins and their relationship to malignant and benign breast tumors. Adv. Prost. Thromb. Res. 1980; 4:595-600.

Bergstrom S. Isolation, structure and actions of prostaglandins. Prostaglandins. 2nd Nobel Symposium, (ed) S. Bergstrom and B. Samuelsson. Almquist and Wiksell Stockholm, 1967.

Berstock D. A., Houghton J., Bennett A. Improved anticancer effect by combining cytotoxic drugs with an inhibitor of prostaglandin synthesis. Adv. Prost. Thromb. Res. 1980; 6:567-69.

Bitonti A. J., Sjoerdsma A., McCann P. P., et al. Reversal of chloroquine resistance in malaria parasite Plasmodium falciparum by desipramine. Science 1988; 242:1301-03.

Borglum J. D., Pedersen S. B., Ailhaud G., et al. Differential expression of prostaglandin receptor mRNAs during adipose cell differentiation. Prostaglandins Other Lipid Mediat. 1999; 57:305-17.

Bottomley A. Depression in cancer patients: A literature review. Eur. J. Cancer Care (Engl) 1998; 7(3):181-91.

Breau J. L., Morere J. F., Israel L. Regression and the slowing of growth of human pulmonary metastases induced by piroxicam, an inhibitor of prostaglandin synthesis. Bull Cancer 1989; 76:321-28.

Breitbart, W. Psychotropic adjuvant analgesics for pain in cancer and AIDS Psychooncology 1998; 7(4):333-45.

Buda J. A., Suciu-Foca N., Blomain E., McManus S., Reemtsma K. Impaired cell-mediated immunity in patients with cancer. J. Surg. Onc. 1975; 7:25-529.

Cameron D. J., O'Brien P. Relationship of the suppression of macrophage mediated tumor cytotoxicity in conjunction with secretion of prostaglandin from the macrophages of breast cancer patients. Int. J. Immunopharm. 1982; 4(6):445-50.

Cameron D. J., Stromberg B. V. The ability of macrophages from head and neck cancer patients to kill tumor cells. Effects of prostaglandin inhibitors on cytotoxicity. Cancer 1984; 54(11):2403-8.

Chang M. C. J., Grange E., Rabin O., et al. Lithium decreases turnover of arachidonate in several brain phospholipids. Neurosci. Lett. 1996; 230:171-74.

Chan G., Boyle J. O., Yang E. K., Zhang F., Sacks, et al. Cyclooxygenase-2 expression is up-regulated in squamous cell carcinoma of the head and neck. Cancer Res. 1999; 59(5):991-94.

Chiarugi V., Magnelli L., Gallo O. COX-2, iNOS and p53 as play-makers of tumor angiogenesis (review). Int. J. Mol. Med. 1998; 2(6):715-0.

Choudry M. A., Uddin S., Sayeed M. M. Prostaglandin E2 modulation of p59fyn tyrosine kinase in T-lymphocytes during sepsis. J. Immunol. 1998; 160(2):929-35.

Cohen L. A., Karmali R. A. Endogenous prostaglandin production by established cultures of neoplastic rat mammary epithelial cells. In Vitro 1984; 20(2):119-26.

Cohen Y., Chetrit A., Cohen Y., Sirota P., Modam B. Cancer morbidity in psychiatric patients: Influence of lithium carbonate treatment. Med. Oncol. 1998; 15(1):32-6.

Colleoni M., Mandala M., Perruzotti G., Robertson C., Bredart A., et al. Depression and degree of acceptance of adjuvant cytotoxic drugs Lancet 2000; 356:1326-27.

Cooper C., Jones H. G., Weller R. O., Walker V. Production of prostaglandins and thromboxane by isolated cells from intracranial tumors. J. Neurol. Neurosurg. Psych. 1984; 47:579-84.

Cotterchio M., Kreiger N., Darlington G., Steingart A. Antidepressant medication use and breast cancer risk. Am. J. Epidemiol. 2000; 151(10):951-57.

Damtew B., Spagnuolo P. J. Tumor cell-endothelial cell interactions: Evidence for roles for lipoxygenase products of arachidonic acid in metastasis. Prostaglandins Leukot. Essential Fatty Acids 1978; 56(4):295-300.

Daniel L. W., Sciorra V. A., Ghosh S. Phospholipase D, tumor promoters, proliferation and prostaglandins. Biochim. Biophys. Acta. 1999;1439(2):265-76.

Daniel T. O., Liu H., Morrow J. D., Crews B. C., Marnett L. J. Thromboxane A2 is a mediator of cyclooxygenase dependent endothelial migration and angiogenesis. Cancer Res. 1999; 59(18):4574-753.

Di Battista J. A., Martel-Pelletier J., Pelletier J. Suppression of tumor necrosis factor (TNF alpha)gene expression by prostaglandin E2. Role of early growth response protein-1(Egr-1). Osteoarthritis Cartilage 1999; 7(4):395-98.

Dilman V. R. Metabolic immunosuppression which increases the risk of cancer. Lancet II 1977; 1207-10.

Dittmann K. H., Mayer C., Rodemann H. P. et al. MK-886, a leukotriene biosynthesis inhibitor, induces antiproliferative effects and apoptosis in HL-60 cells. Leuk. Res. 1998; 22:49-53.

Dore-Duffy P. Differential effect of prostaglandins and other products of arachidonic acid metabolism on measles virus replication in vero cells. Prosta. Leuk. Med. 1982; 8:73-82.

Duffy C. P., Elliott C. J., O'Connor R. A., Heenan M. M., Coyle S., et al. Enhancement of chemotherapeutic drug toxicity to human tumor cells in vitro by a subset of non-steroidal anti-inflammatory drugs (NSAIDs). Eur. J. Cancer 1998; 34(8):1250-9.

Eckmann L., Stenson W. F., Savidge T. C., et al. Role of intestinal epithelial cells in the host secretory response to infection by invasive bacteria. Bacterial entry induces epithelial prostaglandin h synthase-2 expression and prostaglandin E2 and F2 alpha production. J. Clin. Invest. 1997; 100:296-309.

Ellis E. F., Rosenblum W. I., Birkle D. L. Lowering of brain levels of the depressant prostaglandin D2 by the antidepressant tranylcypromine. Biochem. Pharmacol. 1982; 31:1783-84.

Emond V., Fortier M. A., Murphy B. D., Lambert R. D. Prostaglandin E2 regulates both interleukin-2 and granulocyte-macrophage colony -stimulating factor gene expression in bovine lymphocytes. Biol. Reprod. 1998; 568(1):143-51.

Fantone J. C., Elgas, L. J., Weinberger L., Varani J. Modulation of tumor cell adherence by prostaglandins. Oncology 1983; 40:421-26.

Fernandez-Cruz E., Gelpi E., Longo N., et al. Increased synthesis and production of prostaglandin E2 by monocytes of drug addicts with AIDS. AIDS 1989; 3:91-6.

Fiedler L., Zahradnik H. P., Schlegel G. Perioperative behavior of prostaglandin E2 and 13,14 dihydro-15-keto-prostaglandin F2 alpha in serum of bronchial carcinoma patients. Adv. Prost. Thromb. Res. 1980; 585-86.

Fitzgerald J, Edietz T. J., Hughes-Fulford M. Prostaglandin E2-induced up-regulation of c-fos messenger ribonucleic acid is primarily mediated by 3',5'-cyclic adenosine monophosphate in MC3T3-E1 osteoblasts. Endocrinology 2000; 141(1):291-98.

Fosslien E. Molecular pathology of cyclooxygenase-2 in neoplasia. Ann. Clin. Lab. Sci. 2000; 30(1):3-21.

Fukushima M., Kat M. Antitumor marine icosanoids: Clavulones and punaglandins Adv. Prost. Thromb. and Leuk. Res. 1985; 15:415-18.

Fulton A. M. Inhibition of experimental metastasis with indomethacin: Role of macrophages and natural killer cells. Prostaglandins 1988; 35(3):13-42.

Fulton A. M. Interactions of natural effector cells and prostaglandins in the control of metastasis. JNCI 1987; 78:735-74054.

Fulton, C. The prevalence and detection of psychiatric morbidity in patients with metastatic breast cancer. Eur. J. Cancer Care (Engl) 1998; 7(4):232-39.

Gilhooly E. M., Rose D.P. The association between a mutated ras gene and cyclooxygenase-2 expression in human breast cancer cell lines. Int. J. Oncol. 1999; 15(2):267-70.

Goodlad R. A., Madgwick A. J., Moffatt M. R., et al. Prostaglandins and the dog stomach: Effects of misoprostol on the proportion of mucosa to muscle and on the proportion of different epithelial type cells. Digestion 1990; 45:212-16.

Goodwin J. S., Murphy S., Bankhurst A. D., et al. Prostaglandin-producing suppressor cells in Hodgkin's disease. New Engl. J. Med. 1977; 297:963-68.

Greaves K., Ibbotson K. J., Atkins D., Martin T. J. Prostaglandins as mediators of bone resorption in renal and breast tumors. Clin. Sci. 1980; 58:201-10.

Greenberg D. B., Jonasch E., Gadd M. A., Ryan B. F., Everett J. R. Adjuvant therapy of melanoma with interferon-alpha-2b is associated with mania and bipolar syndrome. Cancer 2000; 89:356-62.

Grunwald G. B., Simmonds M. A., Klein R., Kornguth S. E. Autoimmune basis for visual paraneoplastic syndrome in patients with small-cell lung carcinoma. Lancet; 1:658-61.

Hansell N. Manic illness presenting with physical symptoms. Am. J. Psychiatry 1996; 147:11.

Harvey P. R. C., Kimura L. H., Cripps C., Hokama Y. Distribution of prostaglandins B,E and F series in plasma of cancer patients. J. Med. 1981; 12(6):427-32.

Hermann C., Block C., Geisen C., Haas K., Weber C., et al. Sulindac sulfide inhibits Ras signaling. Oncogene 1998; 17(14):1769-76.

Hong S. H., Carty T., Deykin D. Tranylcypromine and 15-hydroperoxyarachidonate effect arachidonic acid release in addition to inhibition of prostacyclin synthesis in calf aortic endothelial cells. J. Biol. Chem. 1980; 2455(20):9538-40.

Honn K. V., Cicone B., Skoff A. Prostacyclin: A potent antimetastatic agent. Science 1981; 212:1270-72.

Honn K. V., Dunn J. R., Morgan L. R., Bienkowski M., Marnett L. J. Inhibition of DNA synthesis in Harding-Passey melanoma cells by prostaglandins A1 and A2: comparison with chemotherapeutic agents. Biochem. Biophys. Res. Comm. 1979; 87(3):795-801.

Horrobin D. F. *Prostaglandins: Physiology, Pharmacology, and Clinical Significance.* Montreal, Quebec, Canada: Eden Press; 1978.

Horrobin D. F., Mtabaji J. P., Manku M. S., et al. *Lithium as a regulator of hormone-stimulated prostaglandin synthesis.* In: Johnson F. N., Johnson F. *Lithium in Medical Practice.* Baltimore, MD: University Park Press; 1978: 243-63.

Horton E. W. Actions of prostaglandins E1, E2 and E3 on the central nervous system. Brit. J. Pharmacol. 1964; 22:189-92.

Houssiau F. A., Kirkove C., Asherson R. A., Hughes G. R. V., Timothy A. R. Malignant lymphoma in systemic rheumatic diseases. A report of five cases. Clin. Exp. Rheum. 1991 9:515-18.

Hughes-Fulford M. Prostaglandin regulation of gene expression and growth in normal and malignant tissues. Adv. Exp. Med. Biol. 1997; 400 (A):269-78.

Hughes-Fulford M., Wu J., Kato T., Fukushima M. Inhibition of DNA synthesis and cell cycle by prostaglandins independent of cyclic. Adv. Prost. Thromb. Leuk. Res. 1985; 15:401-5.

Hughes-Fulford M., Wu J., Kato T., et al. Inhibition of DNA synthesis and cell cycle by prostaglandins independent of cyclic AMP. Adv. Prost. Thromb. Leuk. Res. 1985; 15: 401-4.

Hughes-Wiley M. H., Feingold K. R., Grunfeld C., Quesney-Huneeus V., Wu J. M. Evidence for c-AMP independent inhibition of S-phase DNA by prostaglandins. J. Biol. Chem. 1983; 258(1):491-6.

Isomaki H. A., Hakulinen T., Joutsenlahti U. Excess risk of lymphomas, leukemia and myeloma in patients with rheumatoid arthritis. J. Chronic. Dis. 1978; 31:691-6.

Kalish R. S., Askenase P. W. Molecular mechanisms of CD8+ T cell-mediated delayed hypersensitivity: Implications for allergies, asthma, and autoimmunity. J. Allergy Clin. Immunol. 1999; 103:192-9.

Kaneti J., Thomson M. P., and Reid C. R. Prostaglandin E2 affects the tumor immune response in prostatic cancer. J. Urol. 1981; 126:65-70.

Karmali R. A. Review: Prostaglandins and cancer. Prostaglandins Med. 1980; 5:11-28.

Karmali R. A., Sarkar N. H., Emerson W., Good R. A. Prostaglandin regulation of murine mammary tumor virus production: a basis for some of the glucocorticoid and prolactin actions on mammary tumor cell cultures. Prost. Leuk. Med. 1982; 9:641-55.

Karmali R. A., Welt S., Thaler H. T., Lefevre F. Prostaglandins in breast cancer: relationship to disease stage and hormone status. Br. J. Cancer 1983; 48: 689-96.

Karmali R. A., Horrobin D. F., Ghayur T., Manku M. S., Cunnane T. C., et al. Influence of agents which modulate thromboxane A2 synthesis or action on R 3230AC mammary carcinoma. Cancer Letters 1978; 5:205-8.

Kim J. S., Chae H. D., Joh T. H., et al. Stimulation of human DBH gene expression by prostaglandin E2 in human neuroblastoma SK-N-BE(2)C cells. J. Mol. Neurosci. 1997; 9:143-50.

Koren H. S., Anderson S. J., Fischer D. G., et al. Regulation of human natural killing. I. The role of monocytes, interferon and prostaglandins. J. Immunol. 1981; 127:2007-13.

Kugaya A., Akechi T., Nakano, T., Okamura, H., Shima Y., et al. Successful antidepressant treatment for five terminally ill cancer patients with major depression, suicidal ideation and a desire for death. Support Care Cancer 1999; 7(6):432-36.

Kurzrock R., Lieb C. Biochemical studies of human semen. Actions of semen on the human uterus. Proc. Soc. Exp. Biol. Med. 1930; 28.

Lala P. K., Elkashab, M., Kerbel R. S. W., Parhar, R. S. Cure of human melanoma lung metastases in nude mice with chronic indomethacin therapy combined with multiple rounds of IL-2: characteristics of killer cells generated in situ. Int. Immunol. 1990; 2(12):1149-58.

Lee R. E. The influence of psychotropic drugs on prostaglandin biosynthesis. Prostaglandins 1974; 51:63-8.

Leung K. H., Mihich E. Prostaglandin modulation of development of cell-mediated immunity in culture. Nature 1980; 288:597-600.

Licastro F., Walford R. L. Effects exerted by prostaglandins and indomethacin on the immune response during aging. Gerontology 1986; 32:1-9.

Lieb J. Invisible antivirals. Int. J. Immunopharmacol. 1994; 16:1-5.

Lieb J. Remission of recurrent herpes during therapy with lithium. N. Eng. J. Med. 1979; 301:942.

Lieb J. Remission of rheumatoid arthritis and other disorders of immunity in patients taking monoamine oxidase inhibitors. Int. J. Immunopharmacol. 1983; 5:353-57.

Lieb J. Remission of herpes virus infection and immunopotentiation with lithium carbonate: Inhibition of prostaglandin E1 may explain its antiviral, immunopotentiating and antimanic properties. Biol. Psychiatry 1981; 695-698.

Lieb J. Lithium and immune function. Med. Hypotheses 1987; 23: 73-93.

Lieb J., Karmali R., Horrobin D. Elevated levels of prostaglandin E2 and thromboxane B2 in depression. Prostaglandins Leukot. Med. 1983; 10: 361-67.

Lim J. T., Piazza G. A., Han E. K. et al. Sulindac derivatives inhibit growth and induce apoptosis in human prostate cancer cell lines. Biochem. Pharmacol. 1999; 58: 1097-1107.

Linnoila M., Whorton A. R., Rubinow D. K. CSF prostaglandin levels in depressed and schizophrenic patients. Arch. Gen. Psychiatry 1983; 40: 405-6.

Lofft J. MAO inhibitors. Psychiat Times 1985; 11.

Lupulescu A. Enhancement of carcinogenesis by prostaglandins Nature 1978; 272 (13): 634-36.

Mak O., Chen S. Effects of two antidepressant drugs-imipramine and amitriptyline on the enzyme activity of 15-hydroxyprostaglandin dehydrogenase purified from brain, lung, liver and kidney of mouse. Prog. Lipid Res. 1986; 25:153-5.

Manku M. S., Horrobin D. F. Chloroquine, quinine, procaine, quinidine and clomipramine are prostaglandin agonists and antagonists. Prostaglandins 1976; 12:789-801.

Marks F., Furstenberger G., Muller-Decker K. Metabolic targets of cancer chemoprevention: Interruption of tumor development by inhibition of arachidonic acid metabolism. Recent Results Cancer Res. 1999; 151:45-67.

Marrogi A., Pass H. I., Khan M., Metheny- Barlow I. J., Harris C. C., Gerwin B. I. Human mesothelioma samples overexpress both cyclooxygenase-2 (COX-2) and inducible nitric oxide synthase (NOS2): In vitro antiproliferative effects of a COX-2 inhibitor. Cancer Res. 2000 July 15; 60(14):3696-700.

Matsumoto-Taniura N., Matsumoto K., Nakamira T. Prostaglandin in mouse mammary tumor cells confers invasive growth potential by inducing hepatocyte growth factor in stromal fibroblasts. Br. J. Cancer 1999; 81:194-202.

Matsumoto-Taniura N., Matsumoto K., Nakamura T. Prostaglandin production in mouse mammary tumor cells confers invasive growth potential by inducing hepatocyte growth factor in stromal fibroblasts. Br. J. Cancer 1999 Sep; 81(2):194-202.

Mest H. J., Zehl U., Sziegoleit W., et al. Influence of mental stress on plasma level of prostaglandins, thromboxane B2 and on circulating platelet aggregates in man. Prostaglandins Leukot. Med. 1982; 8:553-63.

Minna J. D., Bunn P.A. Jr. Paraneoplastic syndromes in Devita VT, et al. (ed) *Principles and practices of oncology.* Philadelphia: Lippincott, 1982:1476-517.

Mtabaji J. P., Manku M. S., Horrobin D. F. Actions of the tricyclic antidepressant clomipramine on responses to pressor agents: Interactions with prostaglandin E2 Prostaglandins 1977; 14: 25-32.

Molina M. A., Sitja-Arnau M., Lemoine M. G., Frazier M. L., Sinicrope F. A. Increased cyclooxygenase-2 expression in human pancreatic carcinomas and cell lines: Growth inhibition by nonsteroidal anti-inflammatory drugs. Cancer Res. 1999; 59(17):4356-62.

Moreno J. J. Regulation of arachidonic acid release and prostaglandin formation cell-to-cell adhesive interactions in wound repair. Pflugers. Arch. 1997; 433:351-56.

Murata H., Kawano S., Tsuji S., Tsuji M., Sawaoka H., et al. Cyclooxygenase-2 overexpression enhances lymphatic invasion and metastasis in human gastric carcinoma. Am. J. Gastroenterol. 1999; 94(2):451-5.

Murphy D. L., Donnelly C., Moskowitz J. Inhibition by lithium of prostaglandin E1 and norepinephrine effects on cyclic adenosine monophosphate production in human platelets. Clin. Pharm. Therap. 1973; 15(5):810-5.

Nanji A. A. Thromboxane synthase and organ preference for metastases. N. Eng. J. Med. 1979; 138-9.

Newton A. A. Inhibitors of prostaglandin synthesis as inhibitors of herpes simplex virus replication. Adv. Ophthalmol. 1979; 38:58-63.

Nordenberg J., Fenig E., Landau M., Weizman R., Weizman A. Effects of psychotropic drugs on cell proliferation and differentiation. Biochem. Pharmacol. 1999; 58(8): 1229-36.

Ogilvie, H. The Human Heritage (the Ward Jones lecture, Manchester University). Lancet, July 6th, 1957.

Ohishi K., Ueno R., Nishino S. Increased level of salivary prostaglandins in patients with major depression. Biol. Psychiatry 1988; 23: 326-34.

Penninx B. W., Guralnik J. M., Pahor M., Ferruci L., Cerhan J. R. et al. Chronically depressed mood and cancer risk in older persons. J. Natl. Cancer Inst. 1998; 90(24):1888-93.

Peterson, H. I. Tumor angiogenesis inhibition by prostaglandin synthase inhibitors. Anticancer Research 1986; 6:251-4.

Pfefferbaum-Levine B., Kumor K., Cangir A., Choroszy M., Roseberry E. A. Tricyclic antidepressants for children with cancer. Am. J. Psychiat. 1983; 8:1074-6.

Pinelli E., Poux N., Garren L., et al. Activation of mitogen-activated protein kinase by fumonisin B(1) stimulates cPLA(2) phosphorylation, the arachidonic acid cascade and cAMP production. Carcinogenesis 1999; 20:1683-88.

Pirl W. F., Roth A. J. Diagnosis and treatment of depression in cancer patients Oncology (Huntingt) 1999;13(9): 1293-301.

Plescia O. J., Smith A. H., Grinwich K. Subversion of immune system by tumor cells and role of prostaglandins. Proc. Nat. Acad. Sci. 1975 May; 72(5):1848-51.

Popescu C. Z., The role of prostaglandins in the development of malignant melanoma in hamsters. Prosta. Med. 1981; 7:321-5.

Quia L., Kozoni V., Tsioulias G. J., Koutsos M. I., Hanif R. Selected prostaglandins increase the proliferation of human colon carcinoma cell lines and mouse monocytes in vivo. Biochem. Biophys. Acta. 1995; 1258(2):215-23.

Ramsay R. G., Friend A., Vizantios Y., Freeman R., Sicurella C., et al. Cyclooxygenase-2, a colorectal cancer nonsteroidal anti-inflammatory drug target, is regulated by c-MYB. Cancer Res. 2000; 60(7):1805-9.

Ravischandran D., Cooper A., Johnson C. D. Effect of lithium gamma-linolenate on the growth of experimental human pancreatic carcinoma. Br. J. Surg.: 85(9):1201-5.

Rosenberg L., Palmer J. R., Zauber A. G., Warshauer M. E., Stolley P. D., et al. A hypothesis: Non-steroidal anti-inflammatory drugs reduce the incidence of large-bowel cancer. J. Natl. Cancer Inst. 1991; 83:355-8.

Rosenthal S. H. Does phenelzine relieve aphthous ulcers of the mouth? N. Engl. J. Med. 1984; 311:1442.

Rosenthal S. H., Fitch W. P. The antiherpetic effect of phenelzine. J. Clin. Psychopharmacol. 1987; 7:119.

Salama A., Facer C. A. Desipramine reversal of chloroquine resistance in wild isolates of Plasmodium falciparum. Lancet 1990; 335:164-5.

Samuelsson B. Biosynthesis and metabolism of prostaglandins. Progr. Biochem. Pharmacol. 1967; 3:59-70.

Sawaoka H., Kawano S., Tsuji S., Tsugi M., Sun W., et al. Helicobacter pylori infection induces cyclooxygenase-2 expression in human gastric mucosa. Prosta. Leukot. Essential Fatty Acids 1998; 59(5):313-6.

Schaad N. C., Magistretti P. J., Schorderet M. Prostanoids and their role in cell-cell interactions in the central nervous system. Neurochem. Int 1991; 18(3):303-22.

Sela O., Shoenfeld Y. Cancer and autoimmune diseases. Semin. Arthritis Rheum. 1988; 18:77-87.

Sheng H., Williams C. S., Shao J., Liang P., Dubois R. N., Beauchamp R. D. Induction of cyclooxygenase-2 by activated Ha-ras oncogene in Rat-1 fibroblasts and the role of mutated protein kinase pathway. J. Biol. Chem. 1998; 273(34): 22121-7.

Sinha D., Addya S., Murer E., Boden G. 15-Deoxy-delta (12, 14) prostaglandin J2: a putative endogenous promoter of adipogenesis suppresses the ob gene. Metabolism 1999; 48(6):786-91.

Skinner G. R., Hartley C., Buchan A., et al. The effect of lithium chloride on the replication of herpes simplex virus. Med. Microbiol. Immunol. 1980; 168:139-48.

Stringfellow D. A., Fitzpatrick F. A. Prostaglandin D2 controls pulmonary metastasis of malignant melanoma cells. Nature 1979; 282:76-8.

Taketo M. M. Cyclooxygenase-2 inhibitors in tumorigenesis (part 1). J. Natl. Cancer Inst. 1998; 90(20):1529-36.

Thun M. J., Namboordiri M. M., Heath C. W. Jr. Aspirin use and reduced risk of fatal colon cancer. N. Engl. J. Med. 1991; 325:1593-1956.

Tisdale M. J. Role of prostaglandins in metastatic dissemination of cancer: Minireview on cancer research. Expl. Cell Biol. 1983; 51:250-6.

Villaneuva A., Garcia C., Paules A. B., Vicente M., Megias M. Disruption of the antiproliferative TGF-beta signaling pathways in human pancreatic cancer cells. Oncogene 1998; 17(15):1969-78.

Wahl L. M., Corcoran M. L., Pyle S. W., et al. Human immunodeficiency virus glycoprotein (gp120) induction of monocyte arachidonic acid and interleukin 1. Proc. Natl. Acad. Sci. USA 1989; 86:621-625.

Wang Y. C., Pandey G. M., Mendels J., Frazier A. Effect of lithium on prostaglandin E1 stimulated adenyl cyclase activity of human platelets. Biochem. Pharmacol. 1974; 23: 845-55.

Watkins D. N., Lenzo J. C., Segal A., Garlepp M. J., Thompson P. J. Expression and localization of cyclo-oxygenase isoforms in non-small cell lung cancer. Eur. Resp. J. 1999; 14(2):412-8.

Weinbach E. C., Costa J. L., Wieder S. C. Antidepressant drugs suppress growth of the human pathogenic protozoan Giardia lamblia. Res. Commun. Chem. Pathol. Pharmacol. 1985; 47:145-8.

William C. S., Mann M., Dubois R. N. The role of cyclooxygenases in inflammation, cancer and development. Oncogene 1999; 18(55):7908-16.

Williams E. D., Karim S. M. M., Sandler M. Prostaglandin secretion by medullary carcinoma of the thyroid. Lancet 1968; 1:22-3.

Yoshimura R., Sano H., Masuda C., Kawamura M., Tsubouchi Y. Expression of cyclooxygenase-2 in prostatic carcinoma. Cancer 2000; 89(3):589-96.

Young M. R., Dizer M. Enhancement of immune function and tumor growth inhibition by antibodies against prostaglandin E2. Immunol. Comm. 1983; 12(1):11-23.

Zilberstein D., Dwyer D. M. Antidepressants cause lethal disruption of membrane function in the human protozoan parasite Leishmania. Science 1984; 226: 977-9.

A GIANT STEP FORWARD

"At first people refuse to believe that a strange new thing can be done, then they begin to hope it can be done, then they see it can be done—then it is done and the entire world wonders why it was not done centuries ago."

Francis Hodgson Burnett (*The Secret Garden*)

"Chance favors the prepared mind."

Louis Pasteur

"There is nothing more difficult to carry out, or more dangerous to handle, than to initiate a new order of things...partly from the incredulity of mankind, who do not truly believe in anything new until they have had actual experience of it."

Niccolo Machiavelli (*The Prince*)

***

The Anticancer Properties of Antidepressants: A Synopsis

- Cancer is accelerated replication of abnormal cells.

- Excessive prostaglandin production can create abnormal cells, and accelerate the replication of these cells.

- Prostaglandins self-regulate the chemistry of every cell.

- Excessive prostaglandin production activates all of the putative mechanisms causing cancer.

- Prostaglandins regulate DNA and RNA; the synthesis, inhibition, and expression of genes; and the growth and differentiation of cells.

- Genes determine the variations of cancer—why some people develop lung, others breast cancer.

- Prostaglandin synthesis inhibitors, also known as non-steroidal, anti-inflammatory drugs, can prevent and reverse cancer by inhibiting the cyclooxygenase enzyme (COX-1).

- Cyclooxygenase-2 (COX-2) inhibitors such as Cerabrex also have anticancer actions; it is yet to be shown that they have fewer side effects than COX-1 inhibitors, as was originally claimed.

- Antidepressants block prostaglandins, and accelerate their degradation.

- Depression markedly increases the risk of cancer, as well as accelerating and increasing its mortality.

- More than sixty research teams have shown that antidepressants kill cancer cells (the title of the book is not hyperbole), inhibit their proliferation, protect nonmalignant cells from damage by ionizing radiation and chemotherapy toxicity, convert multidrug resistant cells to sensitive, and target the mitochondria of cancer cells, while sparing those of healthy ones.

- Antidepressants can arrest cancer, even in advanced stages, occasionally reverse it, and significantly extend life.

- Antidepressants kill, or inhibit, the proliferation of the cells of malignancies often resistant to chemotherapy or radiation, such as gliomas, lung, kidney, and liver cancer, resistant lymphomas, and inflammatory breast cancer, with more to follow.

- Cancer is not a hundred diseases, as has been touted, but one disease with a hundred variations.

- Excess production of prostaglandins in the brain depresses mood and immune function, while paradoxically inducing autoimmunity. Prostaglandins cause the diseases; genes cause the variations. A key to future research is the interface between prostaglandins and nucleic acids.

***

In writing this book, I draw on the publications of medical researchers investigating prostaglandins, their role in immune function, cancer, and depression, and the inhibition of these molecules by lithium and antidepressants. Epidemiological studies on the role of depression in predisposing to cancer, and in increasing cancer mortality, were important sources, as were more than sixty articles on the anticancer properties of antidepressants. I am indebted to all of the researchers, not only those whose work I have referenced.

Cancer plagues man and many other species, such as dogs, cats, ferrets, owls, large cats, sea lions, dolphins, beluga whales, catfish, sole, sea turtles, and horses. I will not review what does not cause cancer, but only on what does. I have scant aptitude for methodology, and an aversion to verbosity. A reciprocal relationship between length and significance was first addressed by William of Occam, the originator of "Ockham's Rule" or "Ockham's Razor," five hundred years ago, the aphorism emerging, "The closer to the bone, the sweeter the meat."

People believe that science advances in a slow but steady pace, when in reality long periods of stagnation are followed by radical advances. They tend to believe that major advances are made by "experts" in ivory towers, the pharmaceutical industry, and in government laboratories, and eventually make their way to the bedside, when the traffic is often in the opposite direction; clinical advances are often decades ahead of bench research. Max Planck, Thomas Kuhn, and Paul Feyerabend argued that outsiders often draw into logical relationship facts whose relationship to each other had never been suspected.

We all harbor irrational beliefs, which become delusions when they dominate our thoughts and behavior. We are all vulnerable to brainwashing, with many willing to do the brainwashing. Depressed people tend to be naive, impressionable, relatively easy to manipulate, and to develop cancer, creating inviting targets for con artists, many operating from Madison Avenue. Furthermore, paradigm shifts are often resisted by the guardians of paradigm failures—the anticancer properties of antidepressants conflicting with the cancer cartel. That was to be expected, but not the resistance of cancer patients and their families. I have encountered parents and spouses of terminally ill patients that have been too disbelieving to accept antidepressant therapy for their loved one, even when there was everything to gain and nothing to lose.

The anticancer properties of antidepressants will ultimately alter the perception of cancer, and lessen the dread. They will bring about a substantial reduction in research funding, fewer bankruptcies, fewer patients unable to afford treatment, and a radical reduction in the exploitation of patients with bogus remedies and diets. A less than obvious advantage will be a reduction in energy, water, and landfill use by hospitals.

The current burden of cancer is estimated at $200 billion per year, expected to escalate within the next ten years to $1.5 trillion. In the United States, a single episode of cancer may lead to bankruptcy. In poor, overpopulated countries, those unable to afford hospitalization and standard treatment, are apt to receive rudimentary home care. Safe, effective, inexpensive, and ethical outpatient treatment for cancer would benefit mankind, except those that think nothing of exploiting the misfortunes of others. Few would believe that such treatment is available; this book will show that it is. Antidepressants are not a panacea for cancer, but a major step forward. In the final chapter, I have listed sixty laboratory, clinical, and epidemiological studies on the anticancer properties of antidepressants. If antidepressants are brought into the fold of accepted treatment, chemotherapy, radiation, and surgery will continue to have their roles, but to a lesser degree.

Many factors drew me to studying prostaglandins, including articles authored by David Horrobin. On a Sunday afternoon in the summer of 1980, I traced him to his home in Montreal, and we had a brief telephone conversation. Horrobin was intrigued by my observations of the immunostimulating and antimicrobial properties of lithium and antidepressants, and how they related to his studies on the anti-prostaglandin properties of these agents. In 1977, Horrobin showed that prostaglandins regulate nucleic acids (DNA and RNA).[1] Neglect or suppression of this study has exacted a heavy price. Cancer research has focused on the cell nucleus, with is nucleic acids, and the enzymes and proteins inside the cell, when the cellular contents are regulated by membrane prostaglandins—the membrane far more accessible to therapeutic intervention than the nucleus. Were all of this disseminated and accepted, genomics and biotechnology would not have displaced prostaglandins as prevailing biomedical paradigms. Horrobin lamented that genomics had corrupted any hope of progress in clinical medicine. Time is required to become conversant with prostaglandins, a process similar to learning a new language. Using the wrong language in science and medicine creates major problems.

Horrobin wore many hats, one of which was as an astute philosopher of medicine. In a Lancet essay, he writes, "Most doctors have…lost the sense of the urgency of clinical innovation, have become used to the slow pace of clinical progress during the past 30 years, and have become locked into complacent attitudes that in my opinion are frankly unethical. A culture has developed which stretches right from the family practitioner to the drug regulatory agencies of governments, in which innovation is regarded as suspect and the innovator as someone more likely to harm than to help patients. Their colleagues often pillory those who attempt to innovate clinically…more than anything else; this plethora of negative attitudes is why we are failing to make much progress." In "*Experimental Biology and Medicine*," Horrobin writes, "The escalating costs of the healthcare system will bankrupt both states and individuals. These costs largely arise because we are spending vast

---

1 Horrobin D, Manku MS. Roles of prostaglandins suggested by the prostaglandin agonist/antagonist actions of local anesthetic, anti-arrhythmic, anti-malarial, tricyclic antidepressant and methyl xanthine compounds. Effects on membranes and on nucleic acid function. Med Hypotheses 1977; 3(2):71–86.

amounts on marginally useful treatments that ensure that patients return to the healthcare system again and again. The only way this will change is if we find dramatically effective treatments that remove patients from the healthcare system altogether."

In "*Personal Knowledge*," Michael Polanyi argued that "knowing" is an art, of which the skill of the knower, guided by his personal commitment and his passionate sense of increasing contact with reality, is a logically necessary part. An elderly woman accosted Cardinal Zerah Colburn, a natural calculator, and asked him to explain how he did his astonishing calculations. Colburn responded, "Madam, God put it in my head, and I cannot put it in yours."

Pioneering French physiologist Claude Bernard noted, "I accept specialization in the practice, I reject it utterly in the theory of science." Bernard characterized the ideal biomedical scientist as "interested in everything, alert to the possible major implications of clinical observations, recognizing that the formulation of hypotheses is the beginning of all sound science, willing to devise a hypothesis about everything, yet in the kindest and most tolerant way possible, critical and objective about his observations and those of others, constantly analyzing the validity of facts, whether old or new." A paradigm may fail to emerge not only because of successful opposition, but because no one comes forward to champion it. Thomas Huxley's advocacy of Charles Darwin's theory of natural selection is an exception, not the rule.

NATURE'S MASTER SIGNALERS

"An unbelieved truth can hurt a man much more than a lie. It takes great courage to back truth unacceptable to our times. There's a punishment for it, and it's usually crucifixion."

John Steinbeck (East of Eden)

***

Working at the Columbia University Medical School in the 1920s, obstetrician Raphael Kurzrock noticed that when he attempted artificial insemination, the uterus often expelled the semen. He and Charles Lieb found that human seminal fluid could contract or relax strips of uterine muscle. In an article published in 1930, they remarked that the obstetric history of patients from whom the muscle strips were obtained made their experiments even more intriguing. Uterine muscle from patients with a history of successful pregnancy responded to semen by relaxing, while semen always induced contractions in uterine muscle from women with a history of long-standing sterility.

In the early 1930s, Maurice Goldblatt in England and Ulf von Euler in Sweden showed that factors in the seminal fluid of boars act on various smooth muscles and lower blood pressure. Von Euler named these substances "prostaglandins" because the prostate contains small amounts of them, and he assumed that what he had extracted from semen must have come from the prostate gland. Today we know that every cell in the body, without exception, manufactures prostaglandins or derivates of arachidonic acid. Prostaglandins constitute a physiological response system to any stimulation or stress. They orchestrate cognitive, emotional, behavioral, physiological, pathological, and reproductive responses to the environment. Unlike other hormones, prostaglandins do not travel through the body to influence distant organs, but regulate the cells that produce them and neighboring cells. In examining the Kurzrock and Lieb experiment, one discerns factors in semen and uterine muscle that are so variable as to become paradoxical. These factors are prostaglandins.

At the Karolinska Institute in Stockholm, Sune Bergstrom purified several prostaglandins, determined their chemical structure, and showed that they are formed from essential fatty acids. After collaborating with Bergstrom from 1959-1962 on the structure of prostaglandins, Bengt Samuelsson provided a detailed picture of arachidonic acid and prostaglandin metabolism, and defined the chemical processes involved in their synthesis and breakdown. Samuelsson showed that blood platelets convert arachidonic acid to thromboxanes, while white blood cells convert it to leukotrienes. Thromboxanes constrict blood vessels and cause platelets to clump together and release more clotting factors. This is useful when clotting is necessary to stop bleeding; when this mechanism is overactive, it plays a pivotal role in heart attacks and strokes.

In 1971, John Vane discovered that anti-inflammatory compounds such as aspirin block the formation of prostaglandins and thromboxanes. Vane and Salvador Moncada isolated a prostaglandin in the wall of blood vessels and named it prostacyclin. In dilating blood vessels and inhibiting the aggregation of platelets, prostacyclin opposes the actions of thromboxanes. When prostacyclin is injected into patients suffering from blood vessel constrictions, it often causes depression. For their pioneering research on prostaglandins, Bergstrom, Samuelson, and Vane were awarded the Nobel Prize in Medicine in 1982.

Leukotrienes are involved in the contraction of such smooth muscles as those in the bronchi and bowels, in neuroendocrine transmission, and in the formation of blood cells. They play important roles in asthma and psoriasis. In susceptible people, aspirin and other anti-inflammatory agents can trigger acute attacks of asthma. The cause may be blockade of cyclooxygenase by the anti-inflammatory, diversion of arachidonic acid to the lipoxygenase pathway, and production of an excess of leukotrienes.

The anatomy and function of the cell and the location in the cell of the enzymes that synthesize prostaglandins determines the nature of the end products of arachidonic acid. In cells of the stomach the end products are chiefly prostaglandins; leukotrienes are synthesized primarily in the lungs and white blood cells, to a lesser extent in the skin, bowel and brain. Platelets synthesize thromboxanes. The products of arachidonic acid-prostaglandins, thromboxanes, leukotrienes, prostacyclin, and lipoxins-are collectively referred to as eicosanoids.

Many years ago, researchers believed that prostaglandins self-regulate every cell in the body. I accepted this as a principle, and organized my thinking around it. I concluded that prostaglandins regulate a single master switch inside each cell. Subsequently, I learned that prostaglandins regulate the transport of gases and ions, the functioning of the cytoskeleton (scaffolding) and of such organelles as the Golgi apparatus and mitochondria. They regulate proteins, enzymes, and the nucleic acids that constitute deoxyribonucleic acid (DNA) and ribonucleic acid (RNA). Prostaglandins, and the entities they regulate, often participate in reciprocal feedback relationships. Prostaglandins regulate enzymes and nucleic acids, and enzymes and nucleic acids regulate prostaglandins. Prostaglandins are like minute cogs, orchestrating every component of the functioning of every cell. Prostaglandins are among many chemicals produced by the body, but they regulate the production and response to all of the others. In 1982,

Erik Anggard presciently referred to them as "a generalized physiological control mechanism."

Enzymes

Originally referred to as "ferments," enzymes are proteins that regulate the rate of all chemical reactions in living organisms. There are thousands of enzymes, each with a different chemical structure that determines specific reactions. Enzymes do not invent new reactions, but accelerate the velocity of those already existing. Substrates are molecules upon which enzymes act to produce end products. Measuring about a millionth of an inch, enzymes accelerate chemical reactions to the power of a billion. Without enzymes, fluctuations of temperature and acid-base ratios would eventually convert substrates to end products, but the process would be so slow as to be incompatible with life. Enzymes can generate all of the compounds found in living tissue. They maintain a stable environment inside cells, tissues, and organs despite a changing environment. Some need minute quantities of a coenzyme derived from a vitamin or a mineral.

As animals lack the enzymes to synthesize such fatty acids as linolenic acid and arachidonic acid, they must be supplied by the diet, and are referred to as essential fatty acids. Most of the arachidonic acid supplied by the diet is derived from linolenic acid, a smaller quantity from dietary arachidonic acid. Arachidonic acid is thus derived from three sources; directly from the diet, by conversion from linolenic, acid and from phospholipases acting on membrane phospholipids. Cyclooxygenases converts arachidonic acid to prostaglandins, lipoxygenases convert it to leukotrienes. The enzyme 15-hydroxyprostaglandin dehydrogenase (15-hydroxy) degrades prostaglandins and leukotrienes to end products that are excreted by the lungs. An excess of cyclooxygenase has been recorded in many cancers, a deficiency of 15-hydroxy in others. A reciprocal relationship is suspected in some; more cyclooxygenase, and less 15-hydroxy, would have the net effect of increasing prostaglandin concentrations.

Prostaglandins react to any factor in the environment, internal or external, with which a cell or tissue comes in contact. Optimally, they react physiologically to the stimulus, convey the correct signals to the machinery of the cell, and revert to baseline concentrations. Problems arise when the synthesizing enzymes produce prostaglandins excessively, and cannot restore increased production to baseline. Response to stimuli is distorted, and the tissue or organ may become physiologically or anatomically damaged. In order to function optimally, each cell must control the sequence and rate of enzyme formation. A correct sequence will assure that arachidonic acid is converted to prostaglandins at an optimal rate. Whether prostaglandins are produced within or outside of physiological limits depends more on the activity of enzymes than on the availability of precursors.

Membrane Phospholipids

Every cell is enclosed by an outer membrane and invested by twenty more. Cell membranes consist chiefly of phospholipids (lipids containing phosphorus). Specialized proteins transport fatty acids from the gastrointestinal system to the organs where enzymes and proteins incorporate them into phospholipids. A group of enzymes referred to as phospholipases catalyze phospholipids and liberate arachidonic acid, to be converted into prostaglandins. At least nineteen different phospholipases have been identified.

Anatomy of Prostaglandins

Prostaglandins resemble a hairpin. Each bend bears a carbon atom; side chains containing hydrogen, carbon, and oxygen give each structure its unique form and properties. In consisting of hydrogen, carbon, and oxygen, prostaglandins are referred to as carboxylic acids. Prostaglandins are so miniscule that it was impossible to characterize them and study their metabolic pathways until John Rhyage at the Karolinska combined gas chromatography and mass spectrometry. Contemporary techniques of study include radioimmunoassay, enzyme assay, and photographing enzymes with x-ray crystallography,

Biochemistry of Prostaglandins

Prostaglandins derived from eicosa (20-carbon) fatty acids comprise prostaglandins, thromboxanes, prostacyclin, leukotrienes, and lipoxins. Prostaglandins are synthesized from 20-carbon (eicosanoic) fatty acids such as arachidonic acid. Arachidonic acid is derived from phospholipids in the cell membrane, the essential fatty acid linolenic acid, and directly from arachidonic acid in the diet. Three different eicosanoic fatty acids give rise to three groups of prostaglandins characterized by the number of double bonds in their side chains, for example, prostaglandin E1, prostaglandin E2, and prostaglandin E3.

Prostaglandin synthesis involves the consumption of two molecules of oxygen catalyzed by prostaglandin endoperoxide synthase that consists of cyclooxygenase and peroxidase. Variations in the substituent groups attached to the rings give rise to different types in each series of prostaglandins labeled A, B, and so on. Each cell produces only one type of eicosanoid. In 1991, a gene was isolated that codes for a separate form of cyclooxygenase, cyclooxygenase-2. Cyclooxygenase-1 is referred to a constitutive, as it has clear physiological functions. Cyclooxygenase-2 is induced by inflammatory stimuli in migratory cells and inflamed tissues. Drugs such as Celebrex have highest potency on cyclooxygenase-2 and less effect on cyclooxygenase-1. They have anti-inflammatory effects with perhaps fewer side effects, especially gastrointestinal bleeding. Cyclooxygenase-2 is powerfully expressed in many human cancers, and COX-2 inhibitors may delay the progress of many tumors, or even arrest and reverse them, by causing apoptosis (spontaneous cell death) of tumor cells.

Lipoxygenases insert oxygen into arachidonic acid, giving rise to leukotriene A4, which in turn is metabolized to either leukotriene B4 or leukotriene C4. Leukotriene C4 is metabolized to leukotriene D4 and leukotriene E4. The "slow releasing substance of anaphylaxis" consists of leukotrienes C4, D4, and E4. It constricts the muscles of the bronchial airways, and is a critical factor in asthma. Leukotriene B4 is found in high concentrations in the plaques of psoriasis. Leukotrienes are also involved in regulating reproduction and immunity.

Physiology of Prostaglandins

Prostaglandins exist everywhere in nature—quiet, powerful, and invisible except to X Ray crystallography. Prostaglandins are synthesized by all species from man to insects, shellfish, plants, fungi, algae, sponges, and coral. The membranes, and to a lesser extent the cytoplasm, of every cell produce prostaglandins that self-regulate the cell. Prostaglandins regulate oxygen transport and absorption, carbon dioxide transport and excretion, temperature regulation, calcium metabolism, immune function, acid-base balance, and the synthesis and expression of genes. They regulate heat shock proteins, tumor necrosis factor, chemokines, and cyclic nucleotides. No one has appeared to isolate a physiological process not regulated by prostaglandins. Thus, it is reasonable to infer that prostaglandins synchronously regulate hundreds of other molecules.

Enter "prostaglandins" as a key word in an electronic search of a biomedical database, and you will find thousands of studies revealing their participation in osmosis, immune function, the synthesis of enzymes and proteins, pain, inflammation, wound healing, temperature regulation, metabolism, depression, manic-depressive disorder, insulin and histamine synthesis and release, calcium metabolism, oxygen transportation, urine formation, acid-base balance, digestion, sleep, reproduction, memory, and aging. Prostaglandins regulate the synthesis, activation, release, and degradation of such enzymes as protein kinases. As fatty acids can contribute to the formation of proteins, it is not surprising that prostaglandins regulate the synthesis of DNA, the genetic material of all cellular organisms.

Measured in picograms, or one trillionth of a gram, these miniscule, ephemeral hormones play a cardinal role in, among others, the regulation of temperature, blood pressure, heart rate and rhythm, the clotting of blood, breathing, the production of mucus, and the transport of oxygen from the lungs into the blood. Tears contain small quantities of prostaglandins, whose concentration increases in various eye infections. Tears also contain leukotrienes that markedly increase during attacks of hay fever. A prostaglandin enzyme is key to the promotion of physiological sleep, and high concentrations of prostaglandins can be detected in the spinal fluid of patients with sleeping sickness.

If you are hungry and thinking of food, prostaglandins are playing a role in the brain mechanisms involved. Prostaglandins orchestrate the activities required to obtain and prepare food. They induce the flow of saliva and regulate chewing and swallowing. They mediate the sensation of taste, the perception of hot and cold, and the sight and smell of food. In the abdomen, prostaglandins regulate the secretion of acid in the stomach, the motility of the bowel and the absorption of nutrients and fluids from the bowel. They control the production of bile in the liver, its transport into the duodenum, the secretion of pancreatic fluids and enzymes, and their transport into the duodenum. Prostaglandins regulate the formation of urine, its flow down the ureters into the bladder and its excretion through the urethra. They orchestrate digestion and the elimination of feces.

Prostaglandins play an important role in memory and learning, thus explaining why memory and pain are so closely associated. Post-mortem brains of patients with Alzheimer's disease contain high concentrations of prostaglandins. Chronic use of prostaglandin-synthesis inhibitors such as ibuprofen may reduce the risk of Alzheimer's disease.

Pathology

Abnormal synthesis or metabolism of prostaglandins plays a crucial role in many diseases from the trivial to the deadly. Such disorders and diseases include food intolerance, arthritis, migraine, diabetes, asthma, multiple sclerosis, depression, manic-depressive disorder, hypertension, coronary artery disease, heart failure, strokes, peptic ulcers, ulcerative colitis, irritable bowel syndrome, kidney and gallstones, colic, toxic shock syndrome, disorders of immunity and autoimmunity, and cancer.

Prostaglandin E1 levels are elevated in the platelets in mania and decreased in depression. Prostaglandin E2 is elevated in the plasma, spinal fluid, and saliva in depression. These findings explain why depression predisposes to defective immunity, autoimmunity, and cancer. The elevation of thromboxane B2 in depression explains why that disorder predisposes to heart attacks, high blood pressure, congestive heart failure, and strokes. Depressed gay and bisexual men are 66 percent more likely to contract HIV, and 66 percent more likely to die of AIDS than their cheerful peers. Depression predisposes to Parkinson's disease, asthma, and allergies, migraine, diabetes, osteoporosis, cancer, and Alzheimer's disease. These associations are regarded as interesting but puzzling, as the biological mechanisms appear to be unknown. The missing link is the increased production of prostaglandins in depression.

Whether administered experimentally or induced by ulcerative colitis or cholera, prostaglandins cause abdominal pain and distension, nausea, vomiting, and diarrhea. These observations led Dr. P. D. Buisseret at Guy's Hospital to investigate the role of prostaglandins in gastrointestinal and other more remote symptoms of food intolerance in twelve patients. Prior to the food challenge, each patient had blood drawn for baseline prostaglandin measurement. After the challenge, blood was drawn at intervals to be tested for prostaglandin levels. In each of the cases, the buildup of symptoms correlated with increasing blood levels of prostaglandins. The food challenge was repeated after the patients were given a prostaglandin-inhibiting drug such as ibuprofen or aspirin. In eleven of the twelve patients, there was no increase in prostaglandins, and none of the distressing symptoms. When Dr. Peter Creticios challenged ragweed sensitive volunteers with intranasal pollen grains, the concentrations of leukotrienes in their nasal secretions increased in a dose-dependent fashion. Every substance of abuse tested, among them alcohol, nicotine, marijuana, and cocaine either stimulated or inhibited prostaglandin synthesis. Many pharmacologically active agents paradoxically stimulate and inhibit prostaglandins. Prostaglandins have a key role in withdrawal syndromes, among them the exacerbation of ulcerative colitis that may follow smoking cessation.

Pharmacology

Drugs that halt the synthesis of prostaglandins by inhibiting cyclooxygenase are referred to as non-steroidal anti-inflammatory drugs. The best known are aspirin, ibuprofen, naproxen, indomethacin, and ketoprofen. Cyclooxygenase was characterized in

1976. Although non-steroidal anti-inflammatory drugs reduce pain and inflammation, they have many other "double-duty" uses, thanks to their prostaglandin-inhibiting properties. With chronic use, aspirin can reduce the risk of such cancers as those of the bowel, lung, breast, and ovary.

Chronic low dose use of drugs such as ibuprofen may reduce the risk of Alzheimer's disease. Non-steroidal anti-inflammatory drugs have been used to treat premature labor, renal and gallbladder colic, the skin cancer known as xeroderma pigmentosum, and cystic fibrosis. Non-steroidal anti-inflammatory drugs can prevent recurrences of gallstones. By reversing the spasm of muscles lining the gallbladder, bile ducts, and ureters, non-steroidal anti-inflammatory drugs such as indomethacin may alleviate the colic caused by gallstones and kidney stones, and even facilitate passage of a stone. Many drugs with established mechanisms of action also act on prostaglandins. They include beta-blockers, calcium channel blockers, antibiotics, anti-hypertensives, anti-diabetics, and diuretics.

Signaling

Signaling molecules are small molecules such as prostaglandins, peptides, and proteins, while receptors are surface proteins specific to various signaling molecules. Signal transduction converts extracellular signals into cellular responses. Extracellular signaling molecules are synthesized followed by release and transport to target cells. The signal binds to receptors on the target cell, triggering cellular alteration, and the signal is removed. In endocrine secretion, such hormones as growth and thyroid hormones are released into the blood and target distant cells. In paracrine signaling, the targets are adjacent cells, while in autocrine signaling, the targets are sites on the same cell. Prostaglandins interact with cell surface G-protein coupled receptors.

Clinical Inventories Based on Prostaglandins

If a patient has a mood disorder, his/her prostaglandins are probably not optimally regulated. Proneness to infections and inflammatory disorders are markers for abnormal prostaglandin synthesis or metabolism, as are allergies, asthma, poor healing, periodontitis, diabetes, heart disease, osteoporosis, and cancer. Variation is key to the disorders caused by prostaglandins. Thus, some depressed people are free of infection and autoimmunity, while others are prone to cold sores, shingles, pneumonia, urinary tract infections, rheumatoid arthritis, or multiple sclerosis. It is uncommon to be plagued by defective immunity or autoimmunity and not have an accompanying mood disorder.

References

Abdulla Y., Hamadah K. Effect of ADP on prostaglandin E1 formation in blood platelets from patients with depression, mania and schizophrenia. Br. J. Psychiat. 1975; 127:591-95.

Allen J., Vaughan D., Gillenwater J. The effect of indomethacin on renal blood flow and ureteral pressure in unilateral obstruction in awake dogs. Invest. Urol. 1978; 15:324.

Anggard E. Prostaglandins and related compounds-a general physiological control system. In Holmlund D., Svanvik J. (eds). The treatment of ureteral and biliary pain-a symposium with special reference to the use of indomethacin. Suppl. No.75 Scand. J. Urol. Nephrol. 1982.

Armato U., Andreis P. Prostaglandins of the F series are extremely powerful growth factors for primary neonatal rat hepatocytes. Life Sci. 1983; 33:1745-55.

Arslan A., Zingg H. Regulation of COX-2 gene expression in rat uterus in vivo and in vitro. Prostaglandins 1996; 52(6):463-81.

Atik O., Surat A., Gogus M. Prostaglandin E2-Like activity and senile osteoporosis. Prostagland. Leuko. Med. 1983; 11:15-107.

Bartmann W., Beck U., Lerch H., et al. Luteolytic prostaglandin synthesis and biological activity. Prostaglandins 1979; 17(2):301-11.

Bekemeier H., Geissler A., Vogel E. Influence of mao-inhibitors, neuroleptics, morphine, mescaline, divascan, aconitine, and pyrogenes on prostaglandin-biosynthesis. Pharmacol. Res. Comm. 1977; 9(6):587-95.

Bergstrom S. Isolation, structure and action of prostaglandins. Prostaglandins 21, 2nd Nobel Symposium, ed S. Bergstrom and B. Samuelsson. Alquist & Wiksell, 1967; Stockholm.

Bergstrom S., Carlson L., Weeks J. The prostaglandins: a family of biologically active lipids. Pharmacol. Rev. 1968; 20:1.

Borglum J., Pedersen S., Ailhaud G., et al. Differential expression of prostaglandin receptor mRNAs during adipose cell differentiation. Prostaglandins Other Lipid Mediat. 1999; 57(5-6):305-17.

Borowska A., Mackowiak J., Wisniewski K. Prostaglandins and peristalsis. Prostaglandins Med. 1981; 6:13-16.

Boura A., Boyle L., Sinnathuray T., et al. Release of prostaglandins during contraction of the human umbilical vein on reduction of temperature. Br. J. Pharmac. 1979; 65: 360-62.

Broggini M., Corbetta E., Grossi E., et al. Diclofenac sodium in biliary colic: A double blind trial. Br. Med. 1984; J229.

Buisseret P., Youlten L., Heinzelmann D., et al. Prostaglandin-synthesis inhibitors in prophylaxis of food intolerance. Lancet I 1978; 906-908.

Calvano S., Mark D., Good R., et al. Age-related changes in lymphoid tissue content of prostaglandins in (NZB x NZW) F1 and CBA/H mice. Arthritis Rheum. 1983; 26(1):113-16.

Ceuppens J., Goodwin J. Prostaglandins and the immune response to cancer. (Review) Anticancer Res. 1981; 1:71-78.

Claesson H., Odlander B., Jakobsson P. Leukotriene B4 in the immune system. Int. J. Immunopharmac. 1992; 14(3):441-49.

Collier H., Francis A., McDonald-Gibson W., et al. Inhibition of prostaglandin in biosynthesis by sulphasalazine and its metabolites. Prostaglandins 1976; 11(2):219-25.

Craig G. Prostaglandins in reproductive physiology. Postgraduate Med. J. 1975; 51:74-84.

Creticos P., Peters S., Adkinson N., et al. Peptiede leukotriene release after antigen challenge in patients sensitive to ragweed. N. Engl. J. Med. 1984; 310:1626-30.

Cullen L., Kelly L., Connor S., et al. Selective cyclooxygenase-2 inhibition by nimesulide in man. J. Pharmacol. Experimen. Therapeutics 1998; 287(2):578-82.

Czarnetzki B., Thiele T., Rosenbach T. Immunoreactive leukotrienes in nettle plants (Urtica urens). Int. Arch. Allergy Appl. Immunol. 1990; 91:43-46.

Czarnetzki B., Thiele T., Rrosenbach T. Evidence of leukotrienes in animal venoms. J. Allerg. Clin. Immunol. 1990; 85(2):505-9.

Denzlinger C., Rapp S., Hagmann W., et al. Leukotrienes as mediators in tissue trauma. Science 1985; 230:330-32.

DeWitt D. Prostaglandin endoperoxide synthase: Regulation of enzyme expression. Lipids and Lipid Metabolism 1991; 1083(2):121.

Dhir S., Garg S., Sharma Y., et al. Prostaglandins in human tears. Amer. J. Opthalmology 1979; 87:403-4.

Dore-Duffy P. Differential effect of prostaglandins and other products of arachidonic acid metabolism on measles virus replication in vivo cells. Prostagland. Leuk. Med. 1982; 8:73-82.

Dressler D., Potter H. _Discovering Enzymes._ New York: Scientific American Library.

Dusting G., Moncada S., Vane J. Prostaglandins, their intermediates and precursors: Caradiovascular actions and regulatory roles in normal and abnormal circulatory systems. Prog. Cardiovasc. Dis. 1979; XXI(6):405-30.

Editorial. Slow-reacting substance of anaphylaxis: Leukotrienes. Lancet 1980; 1226-30.

El Attar T. Prostaglandin E2 in human gingiva in health and disease and its stimulation by female sex steroids. Prostaglandins 1976; 11(2):331-41.

Ellis E., Rosenblum W., Birkle D., et al. Lowering the brain levels of the depressant prostaglandin D2 by the antidepressant tranylcypromine. Biochem. Pharmacol. 1982; 31(9):1783-84.

Ellis E., Rosenblum W., Birkle D., et al. The effect of tranyl-cypromine on levels of 6-keto-pg f2alpha and other prostaglandins in brain and mesentery. Artery 1982; 10(6):454-64.

Fantone J., Elgas L., Weinberger L., et al. Modulation of tumor cell adherence by prostaglandins. Oncology 1983; 40:421-26.

Fenton D. Reversal of male-pattern baldness, hypertrichosis, and accelerated hair and nail growth in patients receiving benoxaprofen. Br. Med. J. 1982; 284:1228-29.

Gerozissis K., Rougeot C., Dray F. Leukotriene C4 is a potent stimulator of LHRH secretion. Eur. J. Pharmacol. 1986; 121:159-60.

Gibb W. The role of prostaglandins in human parturition. Annals Med. 1998; 30(3):235-41.

Goodlad R., Madgwick A., Moffatt M., et al. Prostaglandins and the dog stomach: Effects of misoprostol on the proportion of mucosa to muscle and on the proportion of different epithelial cell types. Digestion 1990; 45:212-16.

Goodwin J., Bromberg S., Staszak C., et al. Effects of physical stress on sensitivity of lymphocytes to inhibition by prostaglandin E2. J. Immunol. 1981; 127:518-22.

Hall G., Kenny A. Role of carbonic anhydrase in bone resorption induced by prostaglandin E2 in vitro. Pharmacology 1985; 30:339-47.

Hanly P., Dobson K., Roberts D., et al. Effect of indomethacin on arterial oxygenation in critically ill patients with severe bacterial pneumonia. Lancet 1987; 351-54.

Hanukoglu I. Prostaglandins as first mediators of stress. N. Eng. J. Med. 1977; 296(24):1414.

Hayaishi O., Matsumura H., Urade Y. Prostaglandin D synthase is the key enzyme in the promotion of physiological sleep. J. Lipid Mediators 1993; 6(1-3):429-32.

Holmes P., Sjogren A., Hamberger L. Prostaglandin-E2 released by pre-implantation human conceptuses. J. Reprod. Immunol. 1990; 17:79-86.

Holmlund S., Sjodin J. Treatment of ureteral colic with intravenous indomethacin. J. Urol. 1978; 676-77.

Hong S., Carty T., Deykin D. Tranylcypromine and 15-hydroperoxyarachidonate affect arachidonic acid release in addition to inhibition of prostacyclin synthesis in calf aortic endothelial cells. J. Biol. Chem. 1983; 225(20):9538-40.

Hood K., Gleeson D., Ruppin D., et al. Prevention of gallstone recurrence by non-steroidal anti-inflammatory drugs. 1988; Lancet II; 1223.

Horrobin D. _Prostaglandins. Physiology. Pharmacology and Clinical Significance._ Montreal: Eden Press, 1978.

Horrobin D. The roles of prostaglandins and prolactin in depression, mania, and schizophrenia. Postgrad. Med. J. 1977; 53(Suppl. 4):160-65.

Horrobin D., Manku M. Roles of prostaglandins suggested by the prostaglandin agonist/antagonist actions of local anesthetic, anti-arrhythmic, anti-malarial, tricyclic antidepressant and methyl xanthine compunds. Effects on membranes and on nucleic acid function. Med Hypotheses 1977 Mar-Apr; 3(2):71-86.

Horrobin D., Manku M., Mtabaji J. A new mechanism of tricyclic antidepressant action. Blockade of prostaglandin-dependent calcium movements. Postgraduate Med. J. 1977; 53(Supp l4):19-23.

Horrobin D., Manku M., Mtabaji J., et al. Action of lithium on the responses of the rat superior mesenteric vascular bed to noradrenaline and prolactin. J. Physiol. 1975; 251:24-25.

Janicke U., Forster W. Effects of imipramine, chlorpromazine and promazine pretreatment on the in vitro prostaglandin biosynthesis of rabbit brain and renal medulla. Pharmacol. Res. Comm. 1977; 9(5):501-7.

Johnston M., Kanalec A., Gordon J. Effects of arachidonic acid and its cyclo-oxygenase and lipoxygenase products on lymphatic vessel contractility in vitro. Prostaglandins 1983; 25(1):85-99.

Karmali R., Horrobin D., Menezes J., et al. The relationship between concentrations of prostaglandin A1, E1, E2 and E2 and rates of cell proliferation. Pharmacological Res. Commun. 1979; 11(1):69.

Kather H., Walter E., Simon B. Prostaglandins and obesity. Lancet 1978; 111.

Kurzrock R., Lieb C. Biochemical studies of human semen. Action of semen on the human uterus. Proc. Soc. Exp. Biol. Med. 1930; 28:268-72.

Lee R. The influence of psychotropic drugs on prostaglandin biosynthesis. Prostaglandins 1974; 5(1):63-8.

Leung K., Mihich E. Prostaglandin modulation of development of cell-mediated immunity in culture. Nature 1980; 288:597-600.

Licastro F., Walford R. Effects exerted by prostaglandins and indomethacin on the immune response during aging. Gerontology 1986; 32:1-9.

Lieb J. Remission of recurrent herpes infection during therapy with lithium. N. Engl. Med. 1979; 301(17):942.

Lieb J. Prostaglandin synthesis inhibitors in prophylaxis of food intolerance. Lancet I 1978; 157.

Lieb J. Immunopotentiation and inhibition of herpes virus activation during therapy with lithium carbonate. Med. Hypotheses 1981; 7:885-90.

Lieb J. Remission of herpes virus infection and immunopotentiation with lithium carbonate: inhibition of prostaglandin E1 synthesis by lithium may explain its antiviral, immunopotentiating, and antimanic properties. Biol. Psychiat. 1981; 695.

Lieb J. Remission of rheumatoid arthritis and other disorders of immunity in patients taking monoamine oxidase inhibitors. Int. J. Immunophamac. 1983; 5(4):353-57.

Lieb J. Invisible antivirals. Int. J. Immunopharm.1994; 16:1, 1-5

Lieb J., Karmali R. The role of prostaglandin E2 in seminal immunosuppression. Prosta. Leuk. and Med. 1985; 17:243-50.

Lieb J., Zeff A. Lithium treatment of chronic cluster headaches. Br. J. Psychiat. 1978; 133: 556-58.

Lieb, J. Eicosanoids: The molecules of evolution. Med.Hypoth 2001; 56(6):686-93.

Lofft J. MAO inhibitors. Psychiat. Times Nov 1985.

Lord J., Ziboh V., Cagle W., et al. Prostaglandins in wound healing: Possible regulation of granulation. Advances Prostaglandin Thrombox. Res. 1980; 7:865-69.

Mackenzie T., Zawada Jr. E., Johnson M., et al. The importance of age on prostaglandin E2 excretion in normal and hypertensive men. Nephron. 1984; 38:178-82.

Mak O., Chen S. Effects of two antidepressant drugs imipramine and amitriptyline on the enzyme activity of 15-hydroxyprostaglandin dehydrogenase purified from brain, lung, liver and kidney of mouse. Prog. Lipid Res. 1986; 25:153-55.

Manku M., Horrobin D. Cloroquine, quinine, procaine, quinidine and tricyclic antidepressants are prostaglandin antagonists. IRCS J. Med. Sci. 1976; 4:349.

Matsummura H., Honda K., Choi W., et al. Evidence that brain prostaglandin E2 is involved in physiological sleep-wake regulation in rats. Neurobiol. 1989; 86:5666-69.

Mtabaji J., Manku M., Horrobin D. Actions of the tricyclic antidepressant clomipramine on responses to pressor agents. Interactions with prostaglandin E2. Prostaglandins 1977; 14(1):125-32.

Mtabaji J., Robinson C., Manku M., et al. Prostaglandin A2 at low rates of infusion restores the antidiuretic effect of vasopressin in lithium-treated rats. J. Endocrinnol. 1977; 73:31-6.

Murphy D., Donnelly C., Moskowitz J. Inhibition by lithium of prostaglandin E1 and norepinephrine effects on cyclic adenosine monophosphate production in human platelets. Clin. Pharmacol. Ther. 1973; 14(5):810-14.

Natochin Y., Shakhmatova E., Komissarchik Y., et al. Prostaglandin-dependent osmotic water permeability of the frog and trout urinary bladder. Comp. Biochem. Physiol. A. Mol. Integr. Physiol. 1998; 121(1):59-66.

Oates J. The 1982 Nobel Prize in physiology or medicine. Science 1982; 218:756-68.

Oates J., Garret M., FitzGerald G., et al. Clinical implications of prostaglandin and thromboxane A2 formation. New Engl. J. Med. 1988; 319(11):689-98.

Oates J., Roberts L., Sweetman B., et al. Metabolism of the prostaglandins and thromboxanes. Advances Prostagl. Thrombox. Res. 1980; 6:35-41.

Pickles V. Prostaglandins in the human endometrium. Intl. J. Fertility 1967; 12(3):335-38.

Plescia O., Smith A., Grinwich K. Subversion of immune system by tumor cells and role of prostaglandins. Proc. Nat. Acad. Sci. USA 1975; 75(5):1848-51.

Reasbeck P., Rice M., Reasbeck J. Double-blind controlled trial of indomethacin as an adjunct to narcotic analgesia after major abdominal surgery. Lancet 1982; 115-18.

Reches A., Benalal D., Weissman B., et al. Inhibition by lithium of prostaglandin E1-sensitive adenylate cyclase in neuroblastoma x glioma hybrid cells: Approach to the attenuation of the opiate withdrawal syndrome. Clin. Neuropharmacol. 1982; 5(4):395-404.

Reines H., Cook J., Halushka P., et al. Plasma thromboxane concentrations are raised in patients dying with septic shock. Lancet II 1982; 174-175.

Samuelsson B. Biosynthesis and metabolism of prostaglandins Progr. Biochem. Pharmacol. 1967; 3:59-70.

Samuelsson B. Leukotrienes: Mediators of immediate hypersensitivity reactions and inflammation. Science 1983; 220:568-75.

Samuelsson B., Borgeat P., Hammarstrom S., et al. Leukotrienes: A new group of biologically active compounds. Adv. Prostagl. Thrombox. Res. 1980; 6:1-18.

Samuelsson B., Sven-Erik D., Lindgren J., et al. Leukotrienes and lipoxins: Structures, biosynthesis, and biological effects. Science 1987; 237:1171-76.

Schaad N., Magistrett P., Schorderet M. Prostanoids and their role in cell-cell interactions in the central nervous system. Neurochem. Int. 1991; 18(5):303-22.

Shenkman L., Borkowsky W., Holzman R., et al. Enhancement of lymphocyte and macrophage function in vitro by lithium chloride. Clin. Immunol. 1978; 10:187-92.

Shenkman L., Borkowsky W., Shopsin B. Lithium as an immunologic adjuvant. Med. Hypotheses 1980; 6:1-6.

Sircar J., Schwender C. Antipsoriatic drugs as inhibitors of soybean lipoxygenase. A possible mode of action. Prostaglandins Leukotrienes Med. 1983; 11:373-80.

Skinner G., Hartley C., Buchan A., et al. The effect of lithium chloride on the replication of herpes simplex virus. Med. Microbiol. Immunol. 1980; 168:139-48.

Szczeklik A. Prostaglandin E2 and aspirin-induced asthma. Lancet 1995; 345:1056.

Tessier-Prigent A., Willems R., Lagarde M., et al. Arachidonic acid induces differentiation of uterine stromal to decidual cells. Eur. J. Cell Biol. 1999; 78(6):398-406.

Vane J.Inhibition of prostaglandin synthesis as a mechanism of action for aspirin-like drugs. Nature New Biol. 1971; 231:232-35.

Vane J. Prostaglandins as mediators of inflammation. Adv. Prostaglandin Thromb. Res. 1976; 2:791-801.

Vaughn D., Swaim S., Milton J. Elevation of thromboxane in pressure wounds. Prostagl. Leuk. Essen. Fatty Acids 1989; 37:45-50.

Von Euler Welcoming address. Dept Physiology Karolinska Institutet, Stockhom, Sweden. Nobel Symposium 2, 1996.

Wallen L., Murai D., Clyman R., et al. Regulation of breathing movements in fetal sheep by prostaglandin E2. Amer. Physiological Soc. 1986; 526-31.

Wang Y., Pandey G., Mendels J., et al. Effect of lithium on prostaglandin E1 stimulated adenylate cyclase activity of human platelets. Biochem. Pharmacol. 1974; 23:245-55.

Webb D., Nowowiejski I. Control of suppressor cell activation via endogenous prostaglandin synthesis: The role of T cells and macrophages. Cell Immuno. 1981; 63:321-28.

Weetman A., McGregor A., Lazarua J., et al. The enhancement of immunoglobulin synthesis by human lymphocytes with lithium. Clin. Immunol. 1982; 22:400-407.

DEFEATING CANCER WITH ANTIDEPRESSANTS

Prostaglandins are ephemeral, infinitesimal signalers self-regulating every cell in the body, including those subservient to mood and immunity. Initially perceived as master switches, they are now known to regulate every individual component of cellular anatomy and physiology, including the organelles, cytoskeleton, proteins, enzymes, nucleic acids, and mitochondria. Prostaglandins are responsible, paradoxically, for cell function and dysfunction. When prostaglandin production is correctly regulated, our physiology is healthy. Excessive prostaglandin synthesis induces disease, with genes providing the variations. An ideal anticancer agent would reduce excessive prostaglandin production, so as to shut down the development of cancer. Antidepressants have such properties.

In 2001, I published the first of five reviews on the remarkable anticancer properties of antidepressants. Publishing these articles was delayed by the scientific bigotry and/or conflicts of interest of the editors and reviewers of many cancer, and general medical journals. In 1979, David Horrobin showed that prostaglandins regulate nucleic acids; others later showed that they regulate the synthesis, inhibition, and expression of genes. In 1990, R. A Goodlad showed that prostaglandins regulate cell division, when cancer is accelerated cell division. A therapeutic advance is reinforced when the pharmacological mechanisms are known. In this instance, excessive synthesis of prostaglandins in the brain is known to depresses mood and immune function, and activate the mechanisms of cancer.

The Anti-prostaglandin, Immunostimulating, and Antimicrobial Properties of Lithium and Antidepressants

Depression predisposes, among others, to infection, cancer, osteoporosis, and a host of neurodegenerative, cardiovascular, and autoimmune disorders [1, 2]. Excessive syntheses of prostaglandins is incriminated in all [1, 2]. Lithium and antidepressants have potent anti-prostaglandin, immunostimulating and antimicrobial properties, and antidepressants have the paradoxical ability to mitigate, reverse or induce autoimmunity [1,2].

When synthesized excessively, prostaglandin E2 depresses cellular and humoral immunity, allowing pathogens to replicate [3]. Prostaglandins regulate the physiology, immunity, replication, and toxicity of microorganisms, and the resistance of their hosts [1,2,3,4]. Failure of non-steroidal anti-inflammatory drugs in infectious disorders led to the conclusion that inhibiting prostaglandins has limited value in that context. The prostaglandin-inhibiting properties of lithium and antidepressants have been neglected, [5-10] along with their unique immunopotentiating and antimicrobial actions [2].

In the early nineteen fifties clinicians observed that patients treated for tuberculosis with the monoamine oxidase inhibitors isoniazid and iproniazid experienced elevations of mood and energy. That monoamine oxidase inhibitors have dual anti-tuberculosis and antidepressant properties failed to impact the treatment of infectious disorders. Remission of such manifestations of viral infections as sinusitis, sinobronchitis, frequent colds, sore throats, cold sores, and genital herpes in patients taking lithium carbonate has been reported [11, 12,13]. The polymorphonuclear leukocytes of a twenty-nine year old woman with eczema and recurrent staphylococcal and streptococcal skin infections were unresponsive to standard chemotactic stimuli. Addition of lithium to her polymorphonuclear preparations restored their response.

After receiving lithium carbonate, one gram per day for five weeks she became free of infection and relapsed when lithium was withdrawn [14]. Lithium chloride prevents replication of type 1 and 2 herpes virus in cell culture [15] and augments several in vitro immune reactions [16].

Monoamine oxidase inhibitors can reverse tuberculosis, canker sores, cold sores, genital herpes, upper respiratory tract infections, and plantar warts [17,18,19] Tricyclic antidepressants can reverse aphthous ulcers [20], reduce the frequency of recurrences of shingles[1,2] and remit the pain of this disorder [1,2], prevent post herpetic neuralgia [1,2], destroy leishmania minor and major in vitro [21], and inhibit in vitro the growth of the intestinal parasite giardia lamblia [22]. Tricyclic antidepressants have antimalarial properties; they enhance in vitro susceptibility of plasmodium falciparum to chloroquine, and are lethal in vitro against trypanasoma parasites [23-27]. Selective serotonin reuptake inhibitors can destroy various fungi [28] including candida [29], have antibacterial activity [30], and are synergistic with antibiotics [31].

Impaired lymphocyte function, reduced natural killer cell activity, reduced lymphocyte responses to mitogens, and decreased natural killer cell populations have been demonstrated in depressives [1, 2,32,33]. Tricyclic antidepressants augment natural killer cell activity in vivo and in vitro [34] and the monoamine oxidase inhibitor tranylcypromine enhances defective cell-mediated immunity [35]. As lithium and antidepressants have immuno-potentiating properties, they are effective against a wide range of microorganisms. Evidence to date shows that while lithium has antiviral and antibacterial properties, antidepressants have antiviral, antibacterial, antiparasitic, and fungicidal properties. Response of infection to lithium and antidepressants mirrors that of response to depression, with subjects responding selectively to antidepressants or lithium. Antidepressants are highly specific and humans remarkably variable. Response of depression and infection to lithium or an antidepressant is usually simultaneous, suggesting that the central actions of the drugs are important. While antivirals are not necessarily immunostimulants, lithium and antidepressants are invariably antivirals. If antidepressants double as antibiotics, it would not be surprising if antibiotics doubled as antidepressants, and they can elevate mood to hypomania or mania [36].

Prostaglandins: The Ultimate Cause of Cancer

In 1968, Williams reported high levels of prostaglandins in the thyroid and plasma of patients with medullary cancer of the thyroid [37]. In 1976, Goodwin reported excessive synthesis of prostaglandin E2 in suppressor T-cells of patients with Hodgkin's disease [38]. Numerous studies have confirmed elevated levels of prostaglandins in solid tumors and in the immune cells and body fluids of cancer patients [39, 40]. The isolation of cyclooxygenase-2 (COX-2) [41] and the synthesis of selective COX-2 inhibitors stimulated research into the expression of the enzyme in cancer, and its role in apoptosis. In population studies, chronic use of such prostaglandin inhibitors as aspirin and ibuprofen has reduced the risk of colon cancer by as much as 40 percent [44]. Such conventional prostaglandin-synthesis inhibitors as indomethacin and ibuprofen can arrest and reverse various cancers. Whether to use a prostaglandin-inhibitor, or an antidepressant, is a subject for future research, but I would favor antidepressants first, not the least for their immunostimulating and antimicrobial properties.

Prostaglandins stimulate the synthesis of DNA, and the replication of liver [45] and stomach cells [46]. Other studies have shown a paradoxical, inhibitory effect of prostaglandins on DNA synthesis [47]. Prostaglandins and their synthesizing enzymes are key factors in many signaling events, disruptions of signaling pathways incriminated in many cancers.{48,49] The initiation of metastasis is thought to involve the adherence of circulating tumor cells to endothelial cells or to basement membranes. Prostaglandins and thromboxanes play a role in adherence [49,50], with local thromboxane concentrations possibly determining the sites of metastasis [51]. Immunosuppression is a cause and effect of cancer. Increases in prostaglandins at the primary tumor focus may block surveillance by the immune system, while an increase in plasma prostaglandins may contribute to the suppressive environment for lymphocyte function [52].

In a paradoxical counterpoint to immunosuppression, numerous autoimmune phenomena may occur in patients with cancer [53]. Malignant tumors are diagnosed with increased frequency in patients with such autoimmune disorders as pemphigus, myasthenia gravis, and the Eaton-Lambert syndrome [54, 55]. The paraneoplastic syndrome includes a variety of neurological, hematological, metabolic, cardiovascular, and dermatological disorders, in all of which prostaglandins have been incriminated [55, 56]. As monoamine oxidase inhibitors, originally used in the treatment of tuberculosis, have potent antiviral and immunostimulating properties, it is not surprising that one of them, Matulane (procarbazine), is effective in treating stage III and IV Hodgkin's disease.

Depression: A Precursor of Cancer

In 1998 B. W. J. H. Penninx and her coworkers at the National Institute of Aging provided compelling data for Ogilvie's hypothesis: chronically depressed people over the age of seventy are 88 percent more likely to develop cancer, and 50 percent more likely to die of it than their mellow peers [57,58].

Anticancer Properties of Antidepressants

Many studies show that antidepressants have potent anticancer properties, both in vitro and in vivo, with regard to various antidepressants, mechanisms of action, and cancer cell types. Antidepressants destroy cancer cells, inhibit their proliferation, convert multidrug resistant cells to sensitive, protect nonmalignant cells from damage by ionizing radiation and chemotherapy toxicity, and target the mitochondria of cancer cells while sparing those of healthy ones.[59-78].

The primary prostaglandin-degrading enzyme is highly expressed in normal colon mucosa, but lost in human colon cancers [79,80]. Lack of this enzyme promotes the earliest steps of growth of benign as well as malignant colon tumors [79,80]. When this enzyme was first characterized, every agent tested in the hope of stimulating it either had no effect, or inhibited it. Eventually, researchers showed that amitriptyline and imipramine powerfully activate the enzyme in mice, especially the kidney enzyme, with more than a thousand fold activation by amitriptyline. Amitriptyline and imipramine also had potent activating effects on this enzyme in the brain [81].

Mitochondria, Prostaglandins and Antidepressants

Mitochondria are tiny organelles that supply cellular energy and are involved in signaling, cellular differentiation, control of the cell cycle, growth, and programmed cell death. The cells of malignant gliomas of the brain, and small and non-small cell cancers of the lung, tend to repair DNA-breaks caused by radiation and chemotherapy. In an effort to accomplish cell death by an alternative method, investigators are targeting mitochondria. Small molecule agents known as "mitocans" are able to enter tumor cell mitochondria, reduce oxygen consumption, and activate mechanisms leading to cell death. Agents that can destroy cancer cells in this manner, while leaving normal cells intact, notably include antidepressants [82,83,84]. Laboratory experiments using this approach on various cancer cells, including those of gliomas, are encouraging [65,66]. It goes without saying that prostaglandins are intermediaries between mitocans and mitochondria [85,86,87].

Case Reports

A woman suffering from major depression and advanced liver cancer was treated with psychotherapy, the antidepressant fluvoxamine, glycyrrhizin, acid and dehydroepiandrosterone (DHEA). Various indices of defective immune function normalized, and her liver function tests improved. At follow-up two-and-a-half-years later, she was well and symptom free [88].

In 1990, a 60-year-old woman had a mastectomy for inflammatory breast cancer, followed by excision of infiltration of the chest wall. She was given a prognosis of less than a year. I treated her with various antidepressants, and when relocating in 2003 she was in apparent good health.

A middle-aged man had a two-year history of recurrent glioblastoma multiforme of the cerebellum, resistant to all conventional therapies. Within a week of starting sertraline, he noticed an appreciable reduction in tremor and ataxia. After taking the antidepressant for three weeks, he was virtually free of these symptoms.

Antidepressants can arrest, prevent, reverse, and palliate cancer. Short of that, they have many other uses in cancer care. Antidepressants have potent pain reducing properties, when used alone or in potentiating narcotics. They are a sadly neglected resource in this context, including post-operative pain. .Antidepressants can reduce the severity and frequency of hot flashes in patients treated with chemotherapy for breast cancer, and venlafaxine (Effexor) remits acute neurosensory symptoms secondary to oxaliplatin chemotherapy [89]. The monoamine oxidase inhibitors deprenyl and clorgyline protect nonmalignant human cells from ionizing radiation and chemotherapy toxicity [90], and such antidepressants as nefadazone are capable of reversing chemotherapy-induced vomiting [91].

As the response to antidepressants is highly specific, many patients require multiple trials before responding. Some subjects are refractory to all antidepressants, and some relapse due to tachyphylaxis [92]. Prostaglandins are capable of, paradoxically, inducing pro-and-anticancer actions. The ubiquity of paradox warns that antidepressants are capable of initiating or accelerating cancer. Maintaining an index of suspicion, close clinical observation and limiting the duration of drug trials can mitigate such paradox. Epidemiological studies have failed to confirm the suspicion that antidepressants may induce breast cancer [93]. However, breast cancer has been reported in three men taking selective serotonin reuptake inhibitors [94].

Wherever prostaglandin-synthesizing enzymes convert arachidonic acid or phospholipids to prostaglandins are possible sites of action of antidepressants. By maintaining these enzymes within physiological limits, antidepressants can shut down the mechanisms of carcinogenesis{95]. While lithium has immunostimulating and antimicrobial properties, there is little evidence for its possible anticancer actions. Antidepressants have potent pain-reducing properties, alone or in potentiating narcotics, and considerable potential in post-surgical pain, such as the lingering pain that often follows mastectomy. Antidepressants may enhance sleep, appetite and energy, elevate mood, and mitigate the fear of death. Their immunostimulating and antimicrobial properties are relevant to infection secondary to chemotherapy or radiation.

For various malignancies, combined surgery, radiation, and chemotherapy are not curative; a modest survival benefit is difficult to achieve. Resistant tumors include malignant gliomas, neuroblastomas, and inflammatory breast cancer, cancers of the pancreas, lung, liver, and kidney, malignant melanomas, multiple myelomas, and resistant lymphomas. The propensity of cancer cells to repair breaks caused by DNA-damaging radiation and chemotherapy is thought to cause the resistance, but the antiprostaglandin/anticancer actions of antidepressants and non-steroidal anti-inflammatory drugs suggests otherwise. There is every reason to believe that antidepressants would be effective in childhood cancers, rare cancers, and benign tumors such a desmoids.

Depression increases the mortality, and accelerates the death, of patients with cancer, while antidepressants may extend their lives. The intensity of depression may correlate with the aggressiveness of a tumor. Cancer of the pancreas is noted for its aggressiveness, and for the intensity of depression associated with it, and both could be connected by an unusually high concentration of prostaglandins. Antidepressants can arrest cancer, and reverse it. In combating cancer, clinicians will need a wider selection of antidepressants than currently available. Agencies such as the Food and Drug Administration must begin to view antidepressants as immunostimulants and anti-cancer agents, and develop permissive policies to approve agents with antidepressant properties. The development of biological markers to match antidepressants and subjects would apply to every context in which antidepressants are used. In all likelihood, such markers will involve prostaglandins.

References

1. Lieb J. Remission of rheumatoid arthritis and other disorders of immunity in patients taking with monoamine oxidase inhibitors. Int. J. Immunopharmac. 1983; 3(4):353-7.
2. Lieb J. The immunostimulating and antimicrobial properties of lithium and antidepressants. J. Infection. 2004; 49(2): 88-93.
3. Bankhurst A. The modulation of human natural killer cell activity by prostaglandins. J. Clin. Lab. Immunol. 1982; 7:8591.
4. Lieb J. Antidepressants, eicosanoids and the prevention and treatment of cancer. Plefa. 2001; 65(5&6):233-9.
5. Horrobin D. F., Manku M. S. Roles of xanthine compounds. Effects on membranes and on nucleic acid function.suggested by the actions of local anesthetic, anti-arrhythmic, anti-malarial, tricyclic anti-depressant, and methyl xanthine compounds. Medical Hypotheses 1977; 3(2):71-86.
6. Lee R. The influence of psychotropic drugs on prostaglandin biosynthesis. Prostaglandins 1974; 5(1):63-8.
7. Hong S., Carty T., Deykin D. Tranylcypromine and 15-hydroperoxyarachidonate affect arachidonic acid release in addition to inhibition of prostacyclin synthesis in calf aortic endothelial cells. J. Biol. Chem. 1983; 225(20): 9538-40.
8. Manku M. S., Horrobin D. F. Chloroquine, quinine, procaine, quinidine and clomipramine are prostaglandin agonists and antagonists. Prostaglandins 1976; 12:789-801.
9. Yaron I., Shirazi I., Judovich R., et al. Fluoxetine and amitriptyline inhibit nitric oxide, prostaglandin E2, and hyaluronic acid production in human synovial cells and synovial tissue cultures. Arthritis and Rheumatism 1999; 42(12):2561-68.

10. Ellis E., Rosenblum W., Birkle D., et al. Lowering the brain levels of the depressant prostaglandin D2 by the antidepressant tranylcypromine. Biochem. Pharmacol. 1982; 31(9): 1783-84.

11. Lieb J. Remission of herpes virus infection and immunopotentiation with lithium carbonate: Inhibition of prostaglandin E1 synthesis by lithium may explain its antiviral, immunopotentiating, and anti-manic properties. Biol. Psychiat. 1981; 695-8.

12. Hansell N. Manic illness presenting with physical symptoms. Am. J. Psychiatry 1990; 147(11):1575.

13. Amsterdam J., Maislin G., Rybakowski J. A possible antiviral action of lithium carbonate in herpes simplex virus infections. Biol. Psychiat. 1990; 27:447-53.

14. Shenkman L., Borkowsky W., Shopsin B. Lithium as an immunologic adjuvant. Med. Hypoth. 1980; 6:1-6.

15. Skinner G., Hartley C., Buchan A., et al. The effect of lithium chloride on the replication of herpes simplex virus. Med. Microbiol. Immunol. 1980; 168:139-48.

16. Weetman A., McGregor A., Lazarua J., et al. The enhancement of immunoglobulin synthesis by human lymphocytes with lithium. Clin. Immunol. 1982; 22:400-7.

17. Lieb J. Invisible antivirals. Int. J. Immunopharmac. 1984;16(1):1-5.

18. Rosenthal S., Fitch W. The antiherpetic effects of phenelzine. J. Clin. Psychopharmac. 1987; 7(2):119.

19. Lofft J. MAO inhibitors. Psychiat. Times Nov, 1985.

20. Yeragani V., Phol R., Keshavan, M., et al. Are tricyclic antidepressants effective for aphthous ulcers? J. Clin. Psychiat. 1987; 48(6):256.

21. Zilberstein D., Dwyer D. Antidepressants cause lethal disruption of membrane function in the human protozoan parasite leishmania. Science 1984; 226:977.

22. Weinbach E., Costa J., Wieder S., Antidepressant drugs suppress growth of the human pathogenic protozoan giardia lamblia. Res. Commun. Chem. Pathol. Pharm. 1985; 47(1):145-8.

23. Bitionti A., Sjoerdsma A., McCann P., et al. Reversal of chloroquine resistance in malaria parasite plasmodium falciparum by desipramine. Science 1998; 242(48883):1301-3.

24. Salama A., Facer C. Desipramine reversal of chloroquine resistance in wild isolates of plasmodium falciparum. Lancet 1990; 335:164-5.

25. Dutta P., Pinto J., Rivlin R. Antimalarial properties of imipramine and amitriptyline. J. Protozool. 1990; 37(1): 54-8.

26. Coutaux A., Mooney J., Wirth D. Neuronal monoamine reuptake inhibitors enhance in vitro susceptibility to chloroquine in resistant Plasmodium falciparum. Antimicrob Agents Chemother 1994; 38(6):1419-21.

27. Doyle P., Weinbach E. The activity of tricyclic antidepressant drugs against Trypanosoma cruzi. Exp. Parasitol. 1989; 68(2):230-4.

28. Lass—Florl C., Dierich M. P., Fuchs D., et al. Antifungal activity against Candida species by the selective serotonin reuptake inhibitor sertraline. Clin. Infect. Dis. 2001; 33(12):E135-6.

29. Lass-Florl C., Dierich M., Fuchs D., et al. Antifungal properties of selective serotonin reuptake inhibitors against aspergillus species in vitro. J. Antimicrob. Chemother. 2001; 48(b):775-9.

30. Munoz-Bellido J., Munoz-Criado S., Garcia-Rodriguez J. Antimicrobial activity of psychotropic drugs: selective serotonin reuptake inhibitors. Int. J. Antimicrob. Agents 2000; 14(3):177-80.

31. Munoz-Bellido J., Munoz-Criado S., Garcia-Rodriguez J. In-vitro activity of psychiatric drugs against Corynebacterium

unrealyticum (Corynebacterium group D2). J. Antimicrob. Chemother. 1996; 37(5):1005-9.

32. Calabrese J., Skwerer R., Barna B., et al. Depression, immunocompetence, and prostaglandins of the E series. Psychiat. Res. 1984; 17:41-7.

33. Evans D. L, Pedersen C. A, and Folds J. D. Major depression and immunity: Preliminary evidence of decreased natural killer cell populations. Prog. Neurol. Psychopharmacol. Biol. Psychiat. 1988; 12:739-74.

34. Frank M., Hendricks S., and Johnson D., et al. Antidepressants augments natural killer cell activity: In vivo and in vitro. Neuropsychobiology 1999; 39(1): 8-24.

35. Leung K., Mihich E. Prostaglandin modulation of development of cell-mediated immunity in culture. Nature 1980; 288:597-660.

36. Abouesh A., Stone C., Hobbs W. Antimicrobial-induced mania (antibiomania): A review of spontaneous reports. J. Clin. Psychopharmacol. 2002; 22(1):71-81.

37. Williams E. D., Karim S. M. M., Sandler M. Prostaglandin secretion by medullary carcinoma of the thyroid. Lancet 1968; 1:22-3.

38. Goodwin J. S., Murphy S., Bankhurst A. D., et al. Prostaglandin-producing suppressor cells in Hodgkin's disease. N. Engl. J. Med. 1977; 297:963-8.

39. Bennett A., Carter R. L., Stamford, I. F., Tanner, N. S. B. Prostaglandin-like material extracted from squamous carcinomas of the head and neck. Br. J. Cancer 1980; 41:204-9.

40. Kokoglu E., Tuter Y., Sandikci K. S., et al. Prostaglandin E2 levels in human brain tumor tissues and arachidonic acid levels in the plasma membrane of human brain tumors. Cancer Lett. 1998; 132(1-2):17-21.

41. Chan G., Boyle J. O., Yang E. K., Zhang F., Sacks P. G., et al. Cyclooxygenase-2 expression is up-regulated in squamous

cell carcinoma of the head and neck. Cancer Res. 1999; 59(5):991-4.

42. Molina M. A., Sitja-Arnau M., Lemoine M. G., Frazier M. L., Sinicrope F. A. Increased cyclooxygenase-2 expression in human pancreatic carcinomas and cell lines: growth inhibition by non-steroidal anti-inflammatory drugs. Cancer Res. 1999; 59(17): 4356-62; 17 (2):179-91.

43. Watkins D. N., Lenzo J. C., Segal A., Garlepp M. J., Thompson P.J. Expression and localization of cyclo-oxygenase isoforms in non-small cell lung cancer. Eur. Resp. J. 1999; 14(2):412-8.

44. Thun M. J., Namboordiri M. M., Heath C. W. Jr. Aspirin use and reduced risk of fatal colon cancer. N. Engl. J. Med. 1991; 325:1593-1956.

45. Armato U., Andreis, P. G. Prostaglandins of the F series are extremely powerful growth factors for primary neonatal rat hepatocytes. Life Sci. 1983; 33:1745-55.

46. Goodlad R. A, Madgwick A. J., Moffatt M. R., et al. Prostaglandins and the dog stomach: Effects of misoprostol on the proportion of mucosa to muscle and on the proportion of different epithelial type cells. Digestion 1990; 45:212-6.

47. Hughes-Fulford, M. Prostaglandin regulation of gene expression and growth in normal and malignant tissues. Adv. Exp. Med. Biol. 1997; 400 (A):269-78.

48. Karmali R. A., Sarkar N. H., Emerson W., Good R. A. Prostaglandin regulation of murine mammary tumor virus production: a basis for some of the glucocorticoid and prolactin actions on mammary tumor cell cultures. Prosta. Leuk. Med. 1982; 9:641-55.

49. Karmali R. A, Welt S., Thaler H. T. and Lefevre F. Prostaglandins in breast cancer: relationship to disease stage and hormone status. Br. J. Cancer 1983; 48:689-96.

50. Tisdale M.J. Role of prostaglandins in metastatic dissemination of cancer: Minireview on cancer research. Expl. Cell Biol. 1983; 51:250-6.

51. Nanji A. A. Thromboxane synthase and organ preference for metastases. N. Eng. J. Med. 1979; 138-9.

52. Dilman V. R. Metabolic immunosuppression which increases the risk of cancer. Lancet II; 1977; 1207-10.

53. Houssiau F. A., Kirkove C., Asherson R. A., Hughes G. R. V., Timothy A. R.. Malignant lymphoma in systemic rheumatic diseases. A report of five cases. Clin. Exp. Rheum. 1991 9:515-8.

54. Sela O., Shoenfeld Y. Cancer and autoimmune diseases. Semin. Arthritis Rheum. 1988; 18:77-87.

55. Isomaki H. A., Hakulinen T., Joutsenlahti U. Excess risk of lymphomas, leukemia and myeloma in patients with rheumatoid arthritis. J. Chronic. Dis. 1978; 31:691-767.

56. Minna J. D., Bunn P. A. Jr. Paraneoplastic syndromes in: Devita VT, et al. (eds). *Principles and Practices of Oncology.* Philadelphia: Lippincott, 1982:1476-51757.

57. Ogilvie, H. The human heritage (the Ward Jones lecture, Manchester University). Lancet, 1957, July 6th.

58. Penninx B. W., Guralnik J. M., Pahor M., et al. Chronically depressed mood and cancer risk in older persons. J. Natl. Cancer Inst. 1998; 90(24):1888-93.

59. Levkovitz Y., Gil-Ad I., Zeidich E., et al. Differential induction of apoptosis by , Santidepressants in glioma and neuroblastoma cell lines: Evidence for p-c-Jun, cytochrome C, and caspase–3 involvement. J. Mol. Neurosci. 2005; 27(1):29-42.

60. Toki S., Donati R. J., Rasenick M. M. Treatment of C6 glioma cells and rats with antidepressant drugs increases the detergent extraction of G (s alpha) from plasma membrane. J. Neurochem. 1999; 73(3):1114-20.

61. Hsu S. S., Huang C. J., Chen J. S., et al. Effect of nortriptyline on intracellular Ca2+ handling and proliferation in human osteosarcoma cells. Basic Clin. Pharmacol. Toxicol. 2004; 95(3):124-30.

62. Hsu S. S., Chen W. C., Lo Y. K., et al. Effect of the antidepressant maprotiline on Ca+ movement and proliferation in human prostate cell lines. Clin. Exp. Pharmacol. Physiol. 2004; 31(7):444-49.

63. Serafeim A., Holder M. J., Grafton G., et al. Selective serotonin reuptake inhibitors directly signal for apoptosis in biopsy-like Burkitt lymphoma cells. Blood 2003; 101(8):3212-9.

64. Freire-Garabal M., Rey-Mendez M., Garcia-Vallejo L. A., et al. Effects of nefadazone on the development of experimentally induced tumors in stressed rodents. Psychopharmacology (Berl) 2004; 176(3-4):233-8.

65. Freire-Garabal M., Nunez M. J., Pereiro D., et al. Effects of fluoxetine on the development of lung metastases induced by operative stress in rats. Life Sci. 1998; 63(2): PL31-8.

66. Honda T., Favalaro F. G. Jr, Kjanosik T., et al. Efficient synthesis of (-) and (+)-tricyclic compounds with enone functionalities in rings A and C. A novel class of orally active anti-inflammatory and chemopreventive agents. Org. Biomol. Chem. 2003; 1(24):4384-91.

67. Arimochi H., Morita K. Characterization of cytotoxic actions of tricyclic antidepressants on human HT29 colon carcinoma cells. Eur. J. Pharmacol. 2006; 541(1-2):17-23.

68. Daley E., Wilkie D., Loesch A., Hargreaves I. P., Kendall D. A., Pilkington G. J., Bates T. E. Chlorimipramine: A novel anticancer agent with a mitochondrial target. Biochem. Biophys. Res. Commun. 2005; 328(2):623-32.

69. Ballin A., Gershon V., Brener J., Weizman A., Meytes D. The antidepressant fluvoxamine increases natural killer cell counts in cancer patients. Isr. J. Med. Sci. 1997; 33(11):720-3.

70. Varga A., Nugel H., Baehr R., et al. Reversal of multidrug resistance by amitriptyline in vitro. Anticancer Res. 1996; 1:209-11.

71. Sauter C. Cytostatic activity of commonly used tricyclic antidepressants. Oncology 1989; 46(3):155-7.

72. Spanova A., Kovaru H., Lisa V., Lukasova E., Rittich B. Estimation of apoptosis in C6 glioma cells treated with antidepressants. Physiol. Res. 1997; 46(2):161-4.

73. Snyder S. W., Egorin M. J., Zuhowski E. G., Schimpff E. C., Callery P. S. Effects of the monoamine oxidase inhibitor, tranylcypromine, on induction of HL60 differentiation by hexamethylene bisacetamide and N-acetyl-1.6-diaminohexane. Cancer Commun.1990; 2(7):231-61.

74. Volpe D. A., Ellison C. D., Parchment R. E., Grieshaber C. K., Faustino P.J. Effects of amitriptyline and fluoxetine upon the in vitro proliferation of tumor cell lines. J. Exp. Ther. Oncol. 2003; 3(4):169-84.

75. Seymour C. B., Mothersill C., Mooney R., Moriarty M., Tipton K. F. Monoamine oxidase inhibitors l-deprenyl and clorgyline protect nonmalignant human cells from ionizing radiation and chemotherapy toxicity. Br. J. Cancer. 2003; 89(10):1979-86.

76. Xia Z., Bergstrand A., DePierre J. W., Nassberger L. The antidepressants imipramine, clomipramine and citalopram induce apoptosis in human acute myeloid leukemia HL-60 cells via caspase–3 activation. J. Biochem. Mol. Toxicol. 1999; 13(6):338-47.

77. Nordenberg J., Fenig E., Landau M., Weizman R., Weizman A. Effects of psychotropic drugs on cell proliferation and differentiation Biochem. Pharmacol. 1999; 58(8):1229-36.

78. Rosetti M., Frasnelli M., Tesei A., Zoli W., Conti M. Cytotoxicity of different serotonin reuptake inhibitors (SSRIs) against cancer cells. J. Exp. Ther. Oncol. 2006; 6(1):23-9.

79. Yan M., Rerko R. M., Platzer P., et al. 15-Hydroxyprostaglandin dehydrogenase, a COX-2 oncogene antagonist, is a TGF-beta-induced suppressor of human gastrointestinal cancers. Proc. Natl. Acad. Sci. USA 2004; 101(50):17468.

80. Myung S. J., Rerko R. M., Yan M., et al. 15-Hydroxyprostaglandin dehydrogenase is an in vivo suppressor of colon tumorigenesis. Proc. Natl. Acad. Sci. 2006: 103(32):12098-102.

81. Mak O., Chen S. Effects of two antidepressant drugs, imipramine and amitriptyline on the enzyme activity of 15-hydroxyprostaglandin dehydrogenase purified from brain, lung, liver and kidney of mouse. Prog. Lipid. Res. 1986; 25:153-5.

82. Neuzil J., Wang X. F., Dong L. F., Low P., Ralph S. J. Molecular mechanism of "mitocan"- induced apoptosis in cancer cells epitomizes the multiple roles of reactive oxygen species and Bcl family proteins. FEBS Lett. 2006; 580(22):5125-9.

83. Pilkington G. J., Parker K., Murray S. A. Approaches to mitochondrially mediated cancer therapy. Semin. Cancer Biol. 2008; 18(3):226-35.

84. Arimochi H., Morita K. Desipramine induces apoptotic cell death through nonmitochondrial and mitochondrial pathways in different types of human colon carcinoma cells. Pharmacology 2008; 81(2):164-72.

85. Martinez B., Perez-Castillo A., Santos A. The mitochondrial respiratory complex 1 is a target for 15-deoxy-delta12, 14-prostaglandin J2 action. J. Lipid. Res. 2005; 46(4):736-43.

86. Lender A., Shiva S., Levenson A. L, Oh J. Y., Zaragoza C., Johnson M. S., Darley-Usmar V. M. Induction of the permeability transition and cytochrome c release by 15-deoxy-

Delta12-prostaglandin J2 in mitochondria. Biochem. J. 2006; 394(1):185-95.

87. Nencioni A., Lauber K., Grunebach F., Van Pariis,S, Denzlinger C., Wesselborg S., Brossart P. Cyclopentenone prostaglandins induce the mitochondrial lymphocyte apoptosis pathway independent of external death receptor signaling. J. Immunol. 2003; 171(10):5148-56.

88. Jozuka H., Jozuka E., Suzuki M., Takeuchi S., Takatsu Y. Psycho-neuro-immunological treatment of hepatocellular carcinoma with major depression-a single case report. Curr. Med. Res. Opin. 2003; 19(1):59-63.

89. Durand J. P., Brezault C., Goldwasser F. Protection against oxaliplatin acute neurosensory toxicity by venlafaxine. Anticancer Drugs 2003; 14(6):423-5.

90. Seymour C. B., Mothersill C., Mooney R., Moriarty M., Tipton, K. F. Monoamine oxidase inhibitors l-deprenyl and clorgyline protect nonmalignant human cells from ionising radiation and chemotherapy toxicity. Br. J. Cancer 2003; 89(10):1979-86.

91. Khouzam H. R., Monteiro A.J., Gerken M. E. Remission of cancer chemotherapy-induced emesis during antidepressant therapy with nefadazone. Psychosom. Med. 1998: 60.

92. Lieb J., Balter A. Antidepressant tachyphylaxis. Med. Hypoth. 1984; 15:279.

93. Cotterchio M., Kreiger N., Darlington, G., Steingart A. Antidepressant medication use and breast cancer risk. Am. J. Epidemiol. 2000; 151(10):951-7.

94. Wallace W. A., Balsitis M., Harrison B. J. Male breast neoplasia in association with selective serotonin re-uptake inhibitor therapy: a report of three cases. Eur. J. Surg. Oncol. 2001; 27(4):429-31.

95. Lieb, J. The multifaceted value of antidepressants in cancer therapeutics. Eur. J. Cancer 2008; 44:172-4.

CANCER BIBLIOGRAPHY

Antidepressants have pain killing and anti- nausea properties, as well as the ability to remit hot flashes induced by chemotherapy. Their anticancer properties, however, are not widely appreciated. I have assembled a bibliography of studies in which antidepressants were shown to kill cancer cells, inhibit their proliferation, reverse multidrug resistance, protect nonmalignant human cells from damage by radiation and chemotherapy toxicity, and target the mitochondria of cancer cells, while sparing those of healthy ones.

Evidence based, translational, and transformational, are criteria for optimal quality of treatment. The sixty studies listed below fulfill all, and other articles may be retrieved by entering "antidepressants" and "cancer" into Medline or Pubmed. Epidemiological studies have shown that depression predisposes to cancer, and accelerates and increases its mortality. The burden of cancer is estimated at $200 billion per annum, and with our graying population, expected to increase to $1.5 trillion per year within ten years.

Lieb J. Antidepressants, eicosanoids, and the prevention and treatment of cancer. Plefa. 2001; 65(5&6):233-9.

Lieb, J. Antidepressants, prostaglandins and the prevention and treatment of cancer. Med. Hypotheses 2007; 69:684-9.

Lieb, J. "Defeating cancer with antidepressants." ecancermedicalscience. DOI.10. 3332/eCMS.2008.88.

Lieb, J. The multifaceted value of antidepressants in cancer therapeutics. Eur. J. Cancer 2008; 44:172-4.

Reviews

Lieb,J "The remarkable anticancer properties of antidepressants:
DOI.10.3332/eCMS.2008.LTR149

The Cancer Killing Actions of Antidepressants

Abdul M., Logothetis C. J., Hoosein N. M. Growth-inhibitory
effects of serotonin uptake inhibitors on human prostate carcinoma
cell lines. J. Urol. 1995; 154(1):247-50.

Albouz S., Tocque B., Hauw J. J., et al. Tricyclic antidepressant desipramine induces stereospecific opiate binding and lipid
modification in rat glioma C6 cells. Life Sci. 1982; 31(23):
2549-54.

Arimochi H., Morita K. Characterization of cytotoxic actions of
tricyclic antidepressants on human HT29 colon carcinoma cells.
Eur. J. Pharmacol. 2006; 541(1-2):17-23.

Basso A. M., Depiante-Depaoli M., Molina V. A. Chronic variable stress facilitates tumoral growth: Reversal by imipramine
administration. Life Sci. 1992; 50(23):1789-96.

Chou C. T., He S., Jan C. R. Paroxetine-induced apoptosis in
human osteosarcoma cells: Activation of p38 MAP kinase and
caspase-3 pathways without involvement of (Ca2+) elevation.
Toxicol. Appl. Pharmacol. 2007; 218(2):265-73.

Daley E., Wilkie D., Loesch A., Hargreaves I. P., Kendall D. A.,
Pilkington G. J., Bates . . Chlorimipramine: A novel anticancer
agent with a mitochondrial target. . Biophys Res Commun. 2005;
328(2):623-32.

Elojeimy S., Holman D. H., El-Zawahry A., et al. New insights into the use of desipramine as an inhibitor for acid ceramidase. FEBS Lett. 2006; 580(19):4751-6.

Freire-Garabal M., Nunez M. J., Pereiro D., et al. Effects of fluoxetine on the development of lung metastases induced by operative stress in rats. Life Sci. 1998; 63(2):PL31-8.

Freire-Garabal M., Rey-Mendez M., Garcia-Vallejo L. A., et al. Effects of nefadazone on the development of experimentally induced tumors in stressed rodents. Psychopharm. (Berl) 2004; 176(3-4):233-8.

Hisaoka K., Nishida A., Koda T., et al: Antidepressant drug treatments induce glial cell line-derivative neurotrophic factor (GDNF) synthesis and release in rat C6 glioblastoma cells. J. Neurochem. 2001; 79(1):25-34.

Honda T., Favalaro F. G. Jr, Kjanosik T., et al. Efficient synthesis of (-) and (+)-tricyclic compounds with enone functionalities in rings A and C. A novel class of orally active anti-inflammatory and chemopreventive agents. Org. Biomol. Chem. 2003; 1(24):4384-91.

Hsu S. S., Huang C. J., Chen J. S., et al. Effect of nortriptyline on intracellular Ca2+ handling and proliferation in human osteosarcoma cells. Basic Clin. Pharmacol. Toxicol. 2004; 95(3):124-30.

Levkovitz Y., Gil-Ad I., Zeidich E., et al. Differential induction of apoptosis by antidepressants in glioma and neuroblastoma cell lines: Evidence for p-c-Jun, cytochrome C, and caspase–3 involvement. J. Mol. Neurosci. 2005; 27(1):29-42.

Mal'tseva L. F. Effect of serotonin antagonists and monoamine oxidase inhibitors on the antineoplastic effects of serotonin. Farmakol. Toksikol. 1968; 31(6):735-8.

McCormick D. L., Spicer A. M., Hollister J. L. Differential effects of tranylcypromine and imidazole on mammary carcinogenesis on rats fed low and high fat diets. Cancer Res. 1989; 49(12):3168-72.

Pan C. C., Cheng H. H., Huang C. J., et al. The antidepressant mirtazapine induced cytosolic Ca2+ elevation and cytotoxicity in human osteosarcoma cells. Chin. J. Physiol. 2006; 49(6):290-7.

Serafeim A., Holder M. J., Grafton G., et al. Selective serotonin reuptake inhibitors directly signal for apoptosis in biopsy-like Burkitt lymphoma cells. Blood 2003; 101(8): 3212-9.

Snyder S. W., Egorin M. J., Zuhowski E. G., Schimpff E. C., Callery P. S. Effects of the monoamine oxidase inhibitor, tranylcypromine, on induction of HL60 differentiation by hexamethylene bisacetamide and N-acetyl-1.6-diaminohexane. Cancer Commun.1990; 2(7):231-6.

Spanova A., Kovaru H., Lisa V., Lukasova E., Rittich B. Estimation of apoptosis in C6 glioma cells treated with antidepressants. Physiol. Res. 1997; 46(2):161-4.

Tang K. Y., Lu T., Chang C. H., et al. Effects of fluoxetine on intracellular Ca2+ levels in bladder female transitional carcinoma (BFTC) cells. Pharmacol. Res. 2001; 43(5):503-8.

Tocque B., Albouz S., Boutry J. M., Le Saux F., Hauw J. J., Bourdon R., et al. Desipramine eliciits the expression of opiate receptors and sulfogalactosylceramide synthesis in rat C6 glioma cells. J. Neurochem. 1984; 42(4):1101-6.

Toki S., Donati R. J., Rasenick M. M.. Treatment of C6 glioma cells and rats with antidepressant drugs increases the detergent extraction of G (s alpha) from plasma membrane. J. Neurochem. 1999; 73(3):1114-20.

Tsuruo T., Iida H., Nojiri M., Tsukagoshi S., Sakurai Y. Potentiation of chemotherapeutic effect of vincristine in vincristine resistant tumor bearing mice by calmodulin inhibitor clomipramine. J. Pharmacobiodyn. 1983; 6(2):145-7.

Xia Z., Bergstrand A., DePierre J. W., Nassberger L. The antidepressants imipramine, clomipramine and citalopram induce apoptosis in human acute myeloid leukemia HL-60 cells via caspase-3 activation. I Biochem. Mol. Toxicol. 1999; 13(6):338-47.

Inhibition of Cell Proliferation by Antidepressants

Nordenberg J., Fenig E., Landau M., Weizman R., Weizman A. Effects of psychotropic drugs on cell proliferation and differentiation. Biochem. Pharmacol. 1999; 58(8):1229-36.

Sauter C. Cytostatic activity of commonly used tricyclic antidepressants. Oncology 1989; 46(3):155-7.

Stepulak A., Rzeski W., Sifringer M., et al: Fluoxetine inhibits the extracellular signal regulated kinase pathway and suppresses growth of cancer cells. Cancer Biol. Ther. 2008; 7(10):1685-93.

Volpe D. A., Ellison C. D., Parchment R. E., Grieshaber C. K., Faustino P. J. Effects of amitriptyline and fluoxetine upon the in vitro proliferation of tumor cell lines. J. Exp. Ther. Oncol. 2003; 3(4):169-84.

Reversal of Multidrug Resistance by Antidepressants

Peer D., Margalit R. Fluoxetine and reversal of multidrug resistance. Cancer Lett. 2006; 237(2):180-7.

Varga A., Nugel H., Baehr R., et al. Reversal of multidrug resistance by amitriptyline in vitro. Anticancer Res. 1996; 1:209-11.

Mitochondrial Targeting By Antidepressants

Altinoz M. A., Gedikoglu G., Sav A., Ozcan E, Ozdilli K., Bilir A., Del Maestro R. F. Medroprogesterone acetate induces c6 glioma chemosensitization via antidepressant-like lysosomal phospholipidosis/myelinosis in vitro. Int. J. Neurosci. 2007; 117(10):1465-80.

Apoptosis in cancer cells epitomizes the multiple roles of reactive oxygen species and Bcl family proteins. FEBS Lett. 2006; 580(22):5125-9.

Arimochi H., Morita K. Desipramine induces apoptotic cell death through nonmitochondrial and mitochondrial pathways in different types of human colon carcinoma cells. Pharmacology 2008; 81(2):164-72.

Daley E., Wilkie D., Loesch A., Hargreaves I. P., Kendall D. A., Pilkington G. J., Bates T. E. Chlomipramine: A novel anticancer agent with a mitochondrial target. Biochem. Biophys. Res. Commun. 2005; 328(2):623-32.

Fang K. M., Shu W. H., Chang H. C., Mak O. I. Study of prostaglandin receptors in mitochondria of human lung carcinoma cell line A549. Biochem. Soc. Trans. 2004; 32(6):1078-80.

Goovadze V., Orrenius S., Zhivotovsky B. Mitochondria in cancer cells: what is so special about them? Trends Cell Biol. 2008; 18(4):165-73.

Joseph B., Marchetti P., Formstecher P., Kroemer G., Lewensohn R., Zhivtotsky B. Mitochondrial dysfunction is an essential step for killing of non-small cell lung carcinomas resistant to conventional treatment. Oncogene. 2002; 21(1):65-77.

Langbein S., Frederiks W. M., zur Hausen A., Popa J., Lehmann J., Weiss C., Alken P., Cov J. F.. Metastasis is promoted by a bionergetic switch: new targets for progressive renal cell cancer. Int. J. Cancer 2008; 122(11):2422-8.

Lender A., Shiva S., Levenson A. L., Oh J. 15-deoxy-Delta12-prostaglandin J2 in mitochondria. Biochem. J. 2006; 394(1):185-95.

Moreno- Fernandez A. M., Cordero M. D., de Miguel M., Delgado-Rufino M. D., Sanchez-Alacazar J. A., Navas P. Cytotoxic effects of amitriptyline Y, Zaragoza C, Johnson MS, Darley-Usmar VM. Induction of the permeability transition and cytochrome c release by line in human fibroblasts. Toxicology 2008; 243(1&2):51-8.

Nahon E., Israelson A., Abu-Hamad S., Varda S. B. Fluoxetine (Prozac) interaction with the mitochondrial voltage-dependent anion channel and protection against apoptopic cell death. FEBS Lett. 2005; 579(22):5105-10.

Pilkington G. J., Parker K., Murray S. A. Approaches to mito-chondrially mediated cancer therapy. Semin. Cancer Biol. 2008; 18(3):226-35.

Ristow M. Oxidative metabolism in cancer growth. Curr. Opin. Clin. Nutr. Metab. Care. 2006; 9(4):339-45.

Miscellany

Ballin A., Gershon V., Brener J., Weizman A., Meytes D. The antidepressant fluvoxamine increases natural killer cell counts in cancer patients. Isr. J. Med. Sci. 1997; 33(11):720-3.

Penninx B. W., Guralnik J. M. Pahor M., et al. Chronically de-pressed mood and cancer risk in older persons. J. Natl. Cancer Inst. 1998; 90(24):1888-93.

Ronson A. Neurotrophic theories of stress and neurobiology of antidepressants: Applications in psycho-oncology. Bull Cancer 2007; 94(5):431-8.

Steingart A. B., Cotterchio M. Do antidepressants cause, promote or inhibit cancers? J. Clin. Epdemiol. 1995; 48(11):1407-12.

Seymour C. B., Mothersill C., Mooney R., Moriarty M., Tipton K. F. Monoamine oxidase inhibitors l-deprenyl and clorgyline protect nonmalignant human cells from ionizing radiation and chemotherapy toxicity. Br. J. Cancer 2003; 89(10): 1979-86.

Acceleration of Prostaglandin Breakdown by Antidepressants

Mak O., Chen S. Effects of two antidepressant drugs imipramine and amitriptyline on the enzyme activity 15-hydroxyptostaglandin dehydrogenase purified from brain, lung, liver and kidney of mouse. Prog. Lipid. Res. 1986; 25:153-5.

Myung S. J., Rerko R. M., Yan M., et al. 15-hydroxyprostaglandin dehydrogenase as an in vivo suppressor of colon tumorigenesis. Proc. Natl. Acad. Sci. USA 2006; 103(32): 12098-102.

Yan M., Rerko R. M., Platzer P., et al. 15-hydroxyprostaglandin dehydrogenase, a COX-2 oncogene antagonist, is a TGF-beta-induced suppressor of human gastrointestinal cancers. Proc. Natl. Acad. Sci. USA 2004; 101(50):17468-73.

Clinical

Jozuka H., Jozuka E., Suzukei M., Takeuchi S., Takatsu Y. Psycho-neuro-immunological treatment of hepatocellular carcinoma with major depression-a single case report. Curr. Med. Res. Opin. 2003; 19(1):59-63.

Of Historical Interest

(I could not retrieve these articles, but their citations show that the idea of treating cancer with monoamine oxidase inhibitors or tricyclic antidepressants has been around for a long time.)

Branco F. Iproniazid (Marsilid) in cancerology. Arq. Patol. 1959; 31:451-66.

Tettoni E., Sinistrero G. Concerning the effects of a new imino-stilbene derivative (Insidon) in cancer in the course of radiotherapy treatment. Minerva Med. 1963; 54:3898-900.

Uzer Y., Shnider B. I., Gold G. L. A double-blind study with iproniazid in patients with far-advanced cancer. Antibiotic Med. Clin. Ther. 1960; 7:777-81.

EPILOGUE

Max Planck, the originator of quantum physics, argued that advances that are simple, and emanate from unexpected and unanticipated sources are those most likely to be resisted. He believed that the guardians of a failed concept so fiercely oppose a new one that they must literally die in order for a new generation of scientists, not wedded to the dogma, to take over. Many philosophers and historians of science and medicine have echoed his sentiments. In "*Against Method*," Paul Feyerabend notes that suppressing a paradigm, in preference to one politically favored, could permanently damage society. He advised that in the face of rigid old guard resistance, the only recourse to achieve progress might be political intervention. With many politicians now masquerading as doctors, doctors as politicians, and innovators denied access to politicians, that might not work so well today.

Suppression of dissent in medical research and practice, and the brainwashing of nations, would impress the despot of a totalitarian society. With quackery endemic, now amplified by the Internet, and a food industry gone mad with bogus health claims, the man in the street does not know what to believe, and often is unable to differentiate between real and pseudoscience. "Peer review" has become an icon, exploited by the pharmaceutical industry in its advertising, without anyone realizing that it was designed to weed out junk science, and no more. Medicine has stagnated for more than forty years, partially the victim of peer review used by uncreative reviewers and editors to stamp out dissent and innovation. Bruce Charlton has introduced the concept of zombie science, science that died, but was resurrected, often more than once, to serve the self-interest of wealthy, powerful cartels. Some would point a finger at major cancer foundations, which have suppressed the anticancer properties of antidepressants.

Suppression of the paradigm shifts for infectious disorders and cancer has caused tremendous human and economic damage. This book is an appeal to the public to demand their adoption, with as little delay as possible. The anticancer properties of antidepressants could reduce:

The need for hospital beds

Surgery

Surgical equipment

Radiology and equipment

Oncologists

Oncological nurses

Cancer drugs

Cancer journals

Bankruptcies

Patients unable to afford their medications.

Cancer organizations

Cancer meetings and conferences.

Needed funding of cancer research to a fraction of what it is.

Energy and water utilization by hospitals, and their use of landfills

An innovation is like a newborn baby. Unless nurtured, it will not grow to its full potential. In an ethical environment, the innovations for infectious disorders and cancer may well have prevented the health care crisis, or markedly reduced its dimensions. I have witnessed egregious ethical violations in medical schools and hospitals, and by medical and lay media, politicians, and government agencies. Suppression of the anticancer properties of antidepressants by the National Cancer Institute, and the American Cancer Society, sets a new standard for impropriety. Francis Bacon believed that ethics and charity are indispensable in achieving success in science and medicine. While treating humans, we must not forget that cats, dogs, ferrets, owls, and sea lions will not object to receiving antidepressants for their cancers. Why do prostaglandins induce asthma in one person, arthritis in another, cancer in a third, multiple sclerosis in a fourth, and all in a fifth? These variations may be determined by genes, or the location within the cell of the enzymes synthesizing prostaglandins. While excessive production of leukotrienes favors eczema, psoriasis and asthma, and thromboxanes heart disease and stroke, prostaglandin E2 seems to be the chief culprit in cancer.

Imperfections

Matching an antidepressant to a patient may be a time-consuming and stressful period for patient and physician. Of an assumed twenty-five available antidepressants, some patients will respond to ten, others five, yet others one, and some none. Antidepressant folklore holds to considerable inertia before response occurs, thus necessitating trials of weeks or months. In truth, a patient may respond within days or hours.

Antidepressants have side effects, mild, moderate, and rarely life threatening. When a hitherto unknown side effect emerges, one can be sure that "watchdog organizations" create a commotion to pressure the Food and Drug Administration into taking such action as convening a post-marketing surveillance mechanism. Triumphant and virtuous, the drug busters are on the lookout for another victory, never calling for post-marketing surveillance for unexpected, positive side effects that could improve the lives of millions.

Many classes of medication, not the least antidepressants, have paradoxical potential—antidepressants increase or decrease appetite, energy, sleep, libido, anxiety, blood pressure, irritability, suicidality, and homicidality, among others. A few studies allege that antidepressants can increase the risk of cancer, especially breast cancer, while others do not support this assertion. Two studies appeared simultaneously, one alleging that antidepressants inhibit the protective effect of tamoxifen on breast cancer recurrence, the other that they do not. Predictably, the former received tremendous exposure on the Web, the latter almost none, and none of the promoters of the former study published a correction. The irony is that antidepressants have cancer-preventing properties, and some women taking tamoxifen might have been influenced to discontinue their antidepressant. Development of male breast cancer has been reported in three men taking a specific serotonin reuptake inhibitor, and this I find troubling. If you keep paradox in mind, once you have cancer, it is unlikely that an antidepressant will make it worse. It's when you don't have cancer that the risk may exist. The exception might occur in the context of tachyphylaxis.

Tachyphylaxis is a Greek word for the rapid erection of a guard or barrier, pertaining to many classes of medications, including antidepressants. After initially responding to an antidepressant, a patient may relapse within days, weeks, months, or years. It is the bane of antidepressant therapy. Following tachyphylaxis, an equally effective, or even more effective, medication may be identified, after one or many medication trials. Should that fail, the patient may again respond to the original medication, for a brief or extended period. Tachyphylaxis may well be a factor in the treatment of cancer with antidepressants. I suspect that if paradoxical reactions were to occur, they would either be in patients without cancer, or in those developing tachyphylaxis. On balance, people taking an antidepressant for cancer have much to gain, and little to lose.

Depression not responding to antidepressants is referred to as refractory or resistant, and said to be as high as 30 percent. There is no standard definition of what constitutes refractory depression, varying from a single failure to six. My definition is of failing to respond to every available antidepressant, as well as those that may legally be imported. I have treated patients that responded to one antidepressant out of thirty tried. A biological marker to match antidepressant to patient would have substantial humanitarian and economic benefits, and could become a reality if the role of prostaglandins in depression were widely appreciated.

The Paraneoplastic Syndrome

Cancer cells often produce many effects such as pain, fever, loss of appetite, weight loss, wasting, infection, and anemia. Cancer cells may produce hormones that are not controlled by normal physiological control mechanisms. The manifestations include the syndromes of ectopic ACTH, inappropriate secretion of antidiuretic hormone, hypercalcemia, and hypoglycemia.

Neurological disorders include peripheral neuropathy, the Guillaine-Barre syndrome, myasthenia gravis, the Eaton-Lambert syndrome, dementia, and cerebellar deterioration. Blood disorders include low red cell, white cell, and platelet counts. Pigmented lesions, van Recklinghausen's neurofibromatosis, fever, clubbing of the fingers, and rheumatoid arthritis may occur. These pathophysiological effects of cancer are referred to as the paraneoplastic syndrome; prostaglandins are probably causative in all.

Pain

Cancer pain is dreaded, not only because it is common, but also because it is often unrelenting and refractory to pain medications. Cancer pain is invariably attributed to such factors as destruction of tissue, infection, stretching of organs, pressure, or obstruction, but a pivotal role for prostaglandins cannot be doubted. Antidepressants are underutilized in treating cancer pain and cancer surgery pain.

Disclaimer

The information provided here should not be used for diagnosing or treating a medical problem. It is not a substitute for medical care. If you have, or suspect you have a medical problem, you should consult your physician.